CLINICAL ADMINISTRATION
IN AUDIOLOGY AND
SPEECH-LANGUAGE PATHOLOGY

CLINICAL ADMINISTRATION IN AUDIOLOGY AND SPEECH-LANGUAGE PATHOLOGY

Edited by

STEPHEN R. RIZZO, Jr., PhD

Chief, Audiology & Speech Pathology Service
Department of Veterans Affairs
Chillicothe, Ohio

MICHAEL D. TRUDEAU, PhD

Associate Professor
Department of Speech and Hearing Science
Department of Otolaryngology
The Ohio State University
Columbus, Ohio

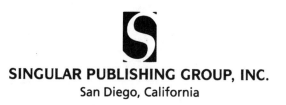

SINGULAR PUBLISHING GROUP, INC.
San Diego, California

Singular Publishing Group, Inc.
4284 41st Street
San Diego, California 92104-1197

© **1994 by Singular Publishing Group, Inc.**

Typeset in 10/12 Palatino by So Cal Graphics
Printed in the United States of America by BookCrafters

Library of Congress Cataloging-in Publication Data

Rizzo, Stephen R.
  Clinical administration audiology and speech-language
  pathology/edited by Stephen R. Rizzo, Jr., Michael D. Trudeau.
     p.   cm.
  Includes bibliographical references and index.
  ISBN 1-56593-088-6
  1. Speech clinics—Administration. 2. Hearing clinics—
Administration   I. Rizzo, Stephen, R.   II.Trudeau, Michael, D.
[DLMN: 1. Practice Management., Medical—organization & adminis-
tration. 2. Audiology—organization & administration. 3. Speech-
Language Pathology—organization & administration. W 80   C6405
1993]
RC247.C45 1993
617.8'0068—dc20
DNLM/DLC
for Library of Congress   93-25798
                                                              CIP

CONTENTS

PREFACE

This book is to be used as a textbook in the education of audiologists and speech-language pathologists (ASLPs), department heads, supervisors, and personnel employed in various health care facilities, hospitals, outpatient clinics, private practices, universities, rehabilitation centers, and other institutions of this type.

This book is written for an introductory course in administration or management. It may be used in courses in which administration, management, supervision, and leadership concepts are studied. No assumption has been made of previous knowledge of these concepts. Although the ingredients are technical in nature, the material is explained in terms that can easily be understood by the reader. This book will assist individuals stepping into administration in understanding the various problems they will face and offers practical advice for the solution of these problems.

Most middle- and lower-level administrative positions, such as department heads and supervisors, are held by health care professionals who have had no formal education or training in administration, management, and supervision. Without going into technical details of these specific positions, this book discusses the managerial aspects common to supervisory positions, whether in ASLP or in any other specialty associated with the health care field.

Experienced administrators can use this material to reevaluate their thinking on contemporary issues in health care from their own perspective and from that of their employees. This text demonstrates to the reader the level of proficiency required to direct individuals in achieving the overall goals of the organization.

The editors realize that the health care workforce consists primarily of women, yet men are actively engaged in the delivery of clinical services. With this in mind, we elected to refer to men and women as supervisors, ASLP administrators, department managers, and similar titles to avoid terms such as he or she, which might prejudice the role that these individuals have in ASLP and in the entire health care field. Furthermore, the use of the term "subordinate" refers to a person whose line/staff position is below that of the supervisor or manager in the department's hierarchy.

We have attempted to provide enough information to make it possible for readers to use these tools with ease at their basic level. It is the editors' hope that readers will subsequently turn to more advanced applications as a result. The creation of this text was inspiring and stimulating as well as demanding and frustrating. We offer you, our readers, the collective work of several highly experienced contributors for your evaluation and reaction.

ACKNOWLEDGMENTS

The foundation of this book represents the result of the first editor's experience with developing an Audiology & Speech Pathology Service from inception. As a result of this experience, valuable insight has been gained, including the insight necessary to develop this book. Special recognition is given to colleagues associated with the Department of Veterans Affairs and to other professionals with whom we have networked over the years.

Editing a multicontributed book requires a great deal of coordination with regard to individual differences and writing styles. The editors thank the contributors for their understanding and cooperation in responding to the demands placed upon them.

For permission to reprint selected material in Chapter 6, the editors wish to thank the following authors, editors, and publisher: Staffing for high productivity by John A. Page and Mark D. McDougall (1988). In M. D. McDougall, R. P. Brandon, V. B. Melton (Eds.), *Productivity and performance management in health care institutions* (pp. 61–82). Chicago, IL: American Hospital Association.

In addition, we would like to thank several librarians who were particularly helpful in searching out materials and providing us easy access to their interlibrary loan resources. Among them are John Package, Merle Alexander, Jennifer Gray, and Daisy Justice of the Department of Veterans Affairs, Chillicothe, Ohio.

Special recognition must be given to Marcy Young, Quality Management Coordinator, Department of Veterans Affairs, Chillicothe, Ohio, for offering substantial creative input in Chapter 5; to Claude Lambert (formerly with the Department of Speech and Hearing Sciences, The Ohio State University, Columbus, Ohio) who provided valuable comments concerning Chapter 3; to Charles Huff, Department of Speech and Hearing Sciences, The Ohio State University, Columbus, Ohio for his review and suggestions for Chapter 7; and to Diana Frame who helped by proofreading Chapter 1.

We would particularly like to thank Joseph E. Rouleau and James L. McNall, JER-JLM Enterprises, Inc., 224 West 2nd Street, Chillicothe, OH 45601, for their thoughtful comments and technical expertise in creating the figure artwork.

We are indebted to Jeffrey L. Danhauer, PhD, Marie Linvill, and the entire staff at Singular Publishing Group for having the vision to realize the need for a text in clinical administration and for their forbearance over the long process of book creation. We would also like to thank John D. Durrant, PhD, University of Pittsburgh Medical Center and The Eye & Ear Hospital, Pittsburgh, Pennsylvania, for providing sample policy and procedure material included in Chapter 2.

Many of the motivational quotations appearing in this book are contained in pocketbooks available through Celebrating Excellence, Inc. 919 Springer Dr., Lombard, IL 60148, (800) 535-2773.

Finally, a special note of gratitude is given to Tracy L. Strawser and David H. Dellinger for their encouragement, support, and constant understanding during the entire time this book was in progress.

DEDICATION

To the students, teachers, clinicians, and researchers of today who will be the clinical administrators of tomorrow. "Do not follow where the path may lead, go instead where there is no path and leave a trail!"

CONTRIBUTORS

David R. Cunningham, PhD
Professor and Director
Division of Communication Disorders
University of Louisville School of Medicine
Health Science Center
Meyers Hall
129 East Broadway
Louisville, Kentucky 40292

Joan Damsey, MA
Chief Executive Officer
Damsey and Associates Ltd.
444 Crawford Street
Portsmouth, Virginia 23704

N. Rock Erekson, MBA
Chief Administrative Officer
University Surgical Associates, P.S.C. (USA)
Childrens Foundation Building
University of Louisville School of Medicine
601 S. Floyd Street
Louisville, Kentucky 40202

Kevin N. Fowler, MS
Business Manager
Lyndhurst Urological Associates
2932 Lyndhurst Avenue
Winston-Salem, North Carolina 27103

Robert T. Frame, DMD, MS
Director, Dental Development Program (113)
Department of Veterans Affairs
810 Vermont Ave NW
Washington, DC 20420

Kenneth W. Heard, PhD
Audiologist, Audiology & Speech Pathology Service (126)
VA Medical Center
4300 W. 7th Street
Little Rock, Arkansas 72205

John A. Page, MS
Executive Director, Health Information Management Systems Society
American Hospital Association
840 N. Lake Shore Drive
Chicago, Illinois 60611

Denise Mill Parker, MBA
Damsey and Associates, Ltd.
444 Crawford Street
Portsmouth, Virginia 23704

David W. Stein, PhD
Associate Professor of Speech-Language Pathology
Division of Speech-Language Pathology and Audiology
Indiana University of Pennsylvania
203 Davis Hall
Indiana, Pennsylvania 15705

Karen G. Stein, MA
Director, Rehabilitation Services
Sewickley Valley Hospital
Blackburn Road
Sewickley, Pennsylvania, 15143

Jay E. Wilkins, BS
Chief, Engineering Service (138)
VA Medical Center
Chillicothe, Ohio 45601.

Cheryl L. Welch, MBA
Chief, Human Resource Management Service (05)
VA Medical Center
Castle Point, New York, 12511

1

FOUNDATIONS OF LEADERSHIP, MANAGEMENT, AND SUPERVISION

*Stephen R. Rizzo, Jr., PhD and
Robert T. Frame, DMD, MS*

"Leaders are like eagles, they don't flock . . . you find them one at a time."

The role of audiologists and speech-language pathologists (ASLPs) in administrative positions has become increasingly complex. As administrators, ASLPs must participate in the planning and monitoring of clinical services, the recruitment of competent staff, and the provision of quality care. They must operate in a system of many interrelated subsystems, including the academic, clinical, and research components of the profession. Most importantly, they must provide leadership. These activities must be performed in a rapidly changing and cost-containment health care environment.

Historically, ASLPs who undertake administrative roles arrive at these positions because of their recognized skills as clinicians, researchers, or teachers; not as administrators. For individuals in administrative positions, their training in ASLP, interpersonal communications, and group dynamics skills have been generally considered attributes. A survey of 125 ASLP university training programs (Rizzo, Gutnick, & Stein, 1992) found that their curricula do not generally provide the management information necessary in today's competitive communication health care environment. Despite the growing awareness of the need for ASLPs to receive training in administration, there is little formal educational training in the areas of planning, human resource management, managing productivity, financial management, marketing, and so forth. The Rizzo et al. (1992) survey supports the need for formal administrative training. Consequently, emerging ASLP administrators often feel unfamiliar with, and are ill-equipped for an administrative role.

This chapter will address some essential leadership, management, and supervisory concepts that are essential to the promotion and support of excellent clinical practice. Although the exact meaning of these titles varies within different institutions, the term "administrator" or "executive" is generally used for top-level management positions, whereas "manager" and "supervisor" usually connote positions within the middle or lower levels of the institutional hierarchy. There are some theoretical differences to consider, but for our purposes the terms "ASLP administrator," "program administrator," "department manager," or "manager" will be used throughout this book. The focus of this chapter will include examination of methods for creating work environments conducive to the development of responsive and innovative clinical practices. The business and health care administration literature that has been developed to encourage the "pursuit of excellence" (Peters, 1982), is a valuable adjunct to this task, and this chapter draws from that body of literature, with discussion, applications, and examples for ASLP health care settings.

LEADERSHIP VERSUS MANAGEMENT

According to Atchison (1990), the essence of leadership can be stated simply as, *leaders have followers.* He explains that *what one does is important only if it motivates positive actions by those who follow.* Atchison concludes with the basic assumption that followers are easy to recognize because they produce more and complain less than others, are proud, not driven solely by pay, and are highly committed to the organization. Because followers have a focus toward the leader's vision, Ross (1986) lists some questions that arise in the minds of emerging administrators.

- Are individuals born with leadership skills or are these skills acquired?
- Can a leader recognize these skills in others?

- What motivates an individual to move into a pattern of leadership?
- Do leaders really function differently from managers?
- Are managers more constrained to operate in terms of tight control and performance?
- Are leaders equally concerned with controls and performance, or do they move from a focus on immediate problems to the larger picture?
- Do they move more easily from the present-day diplomacy to long-range strategic planning?
- Do leaders roll more easily with the punches?
- Are short-range gains forfeited to achieve longer-range goals?
- Do leaders deal more easily with uncertainty and ambiguity?

The trend in health care management has been toward coordinating and integrating human, technical, and other resources to accomplish specific results. Zaleznik (1981) tells us that managers work harder to create structure and, to develop order and progress, they build practices based on precedence and policies. On the other hand, leaders function more by managing by exception than managing by policy and precedence. Leadership encompasses the wise use of power, the ability to envision future goals and directions, vision (a willingness to look beyond the wall), humanism, and practical sense. Flarey (1991) conveys to us that leadership is concerned with goal attainment and task accomplishment, but not at the expense of the people involved. Indeed, leadership is effective only when it draws forth the best in people, is concerned with promoting the general welfare of human beings, and maintains group solidarity.

Simmons and Bixby (1989) point out that leadership is often thought of as charisma, that is, a personal attribute to influence others. Although charisma is, of course, beneficial and assists in peak performance, it is not essential. They point out that what is important is to have a clear grasp of the concepts underlying the leadership process. Leadership is something that can be taught and learned. Although leadership style may be an individual matter formed, to some extent, by individual values and personality, there is a knowledge base and a set of skills which, if understood, are transferable.

To differentiate the concept of management versus leadership it can be said that management focuses on operating the organization, whereas leadership is directed toward giving the effort purpose, meaning, and excitement. Peters (1987) reveals that the challenge is to instill an ongoing sense of newness, intense involvement, focus on quality outcomes, and learning. Some early studies identified two basic leadership styles: (1) *the autocratic style utilizes authority or position power out of concern for tasks or products*; and (2) *the democratic style utilizes personal power out of concern for relationships or people* (Taylor, 1911; McGregor, 1960). These styles were thought to be mutually exclusive (Tannenbaum & Schmidt, 1958), and the democratic style was advanced by proponents of the "human relations" movement as the best, most productive style of leadership (Mayo, 1933). Evidence does indicate that greater production is achievable in organizations that treat employees fairly and as part of a team, and organizations in which participative management is practiced generally outperform others in which a more autocratic, task-centered philosophy exists (Liekert, 1961). However, subsequent research has shown that no single all-purpose leadership style exists (Korman, 1966; Fiedler, 1967). *Successful leaders adapt their behavior to meet the demands of each unique situation* (Hershey & Blanchard, 1982).

THE SHIFT FROM MANAGEMENT TO LEADERSHIP

In recent years, ASLPs have attempted to strengthen their delivery systems by learning from business systems and strengthening their business skills. These concepts have been reinforced by a growing emphasis on accountability, productivity, and their measurement (to be discussed in Chapters 5 and 6). Changing approaches have become available from insights developed in the business world that are even more compatible with ASLP than those previously utilized. Today, the understanding of essential administrative skills is moving to incorporate and elevate leadership skills to a level of major importance. The capacity to develop and sustain a constructive work environment is vital to the ongoing evolution of relevant and high-quality clinical services. The ASLP administrator is responsible for more than the physical resources, the financial base, the business systems, and the mission of the department. The leadership role of the ASLP administrator must be directed toward the human resources within the department as well its impact on the entire health care organization in which it operates. The focus is not so much on tasks as on mission, and on the continuous quality improvement of the effort put forth toward its achievement.

Hickman and Silva (1985) state that to develop an effective winning team, the leader must work in three essential areas: vision, culture, and strategy.

Vision

The administrator must develop a deep concern for the human aspects of management. The leader has the primary responsibility for developing and articulating a vision that guides the efforts of the entire staff. *Vision refers to communication of a dream that gives meaning to daily performance.* This requires an understanding of how things ought to be in the best of all possible situations. *It also requires an ability to assist others to see a new, better, and unknown reality based on the present position.* The vision should be clearly stated so that people understand not only what the effort is leading to in the long run, but also what steps are needed in the present to move in that direction. The vision should be stated in the present tense and should be visible through words and behavior. It can be stated in the form of a phrase, sentence, series of sentences, or a list of vision elements (sometimes called a brag sheet). For example, the ASLP department is committed to the communication health care needs of its clients and strives to improve the delivery of services to meet reasonable expectations.

In sports, world class athletes focus on winning through an intense effort in practice and then develop a strategy to ultimately win in competition. A coach, for example, assists the team to envision itself as winning a national title and, at the same time, assists the team and its members in preparing for particular plays and strategies (Cohen, 1990). In ASLP, this takes the form of the ability to focus professional energy on the purpose and hopes of the work environment. For instance, the delivery of new services for unmet populations can occur quite naturally, as can new methodologies to provide service. In many settings across the country, speech-language pathology services were developed for such patient populations with dementia, head trauma, and dysphagia. In past years, these populations were undifferentiated as specialty groups. Then someone stepped forward and identified them in a new way and assembled others to develop and refine methods for the delivery of services for these groups. These innovations most commonly occur through a leader's vision of clinical practice, knowledge, skills, and methods which can be catalysts for change in light of new insight and understanding.

Hickman and Silva (1985) indicate that vision has several characteristics that give it meaning:

■ It must be visible, something that can be seen clearly in the mind's eye.
■ It must strike at the emotional level; it cannot be just cognitive.
■ It must be stable and enduring, yet capable of change and adaptation.
■ It must focus on quality, not quantity. The focus is on the pursuit of excellence, instead of the need for more resources.

As Peters (1987, p. 435) states, "Developing a vision and, more importantly, living it vigorously are essential elements of leadership." A leader must be prepared to do this in both word and action repeatedly, otherwise the effort tends to drift into mediocrity and the greater vision is lost. People are easily distracted by daily affairs and can feel oppressed and overwhelmed by difficult changes. The vision is most valuable if the leader continues to speak of the vision often. Left in silence, it ceases to have impact and is quickly forgotten.

Culture

The second requirement of leadership is to build and maintain a positive constructive culture within the organization. All human groups have cultures, whether they be nations, social organizations, or work groups. In work settings, these organizational cultures are subject to influence and planned guidance. This is not unlike a family structure which can be modified through positive intervention over time to create a more constructive group. *The elements of the culture include shared values, accepted methods, decision-making styles, communication, and historical background.*

The ASLP administrator's vision of the organization must include more than a service definition and a set of concepts about the relationship of the department to its health care organization; it must also define the culture. The focus must be on both the department and the human elements that comprise the work environment. The traditional management view of administration does not focus on the quality of employee relationships and the nature of the professional interface among colleagues. However, contemporary management (i.e., total quality management, continuous quality improvement, or quality improvement; concepts that will be discussed in Chapter 5) focuses on relationships among staff that are directed toward understanding and guiding them in achieving constructive and creative interactions. Some of the elements of a positive culture that support the "pursuit of excellence" concept include optimism, persistence, fairness, reliability, timeliness, responsive feedback, and a reasonable degree of autonomy for the staff whose opinions are to be respected (Peters, 1987).

Strategy

Hickman and Silva (1985) describe three benefits to be derived from strategic thinking: (1) the need for customer satisfaction; (2) the gain of a substantial advantage over the competition; and (3) the capitalization of company strengths. Applied to the health care environment, these are indeed instructive guidelines. Part of the program administrator's responsibility is to continue to negotiate for key resources such as equipment, staff, and space in order to satisfy the client's expectations. It is vital that the department manager identify the primary needs of the consumer, and plan accordingly to demonstrate the value of the operation in meeting these needs. The best strategy for building excellence within a department is to develop a high-quality practice along with a compelling rationale for the design and purpose of clinical services within a given work setting.

KEY ELEMENTS OF LEADERSHIP AND MANAGEMENT

Several individuals (Cohen, 1990; Ross, 1986; Ziglar, 1986) present some basic principles that can be applied to effective leadership and management:

- Control and time the energy that goes into managing and leading.
- Encourage individuals to develop introspection about their career development.
- Be aware of how individuals can affect an organization's change process.
- Consolidate various activities to determine direction.
- Instill in the staff the concepts of productivity, quality of patient care, innovation, and motivation to get things done.
- Develop a lifelong process of learning, both on and off the job.
- Translate existing facts and information into something innovative, different, or expansive to achieve a solution.
- Learn how to read people, utilizing solid management principles, while applying sensitivity and purpose to meet current expectations.
- Create a work environment for employees that fulfills their need for recognition, achievement, and companionship in order to implement the overall objectives of the department. The better the ASLP administrator performs these duties, the better the departmental results will be.

Ross (1986) points out that whether leadership is different from management is irrelevant, since, in the larger scope of things, true leadership requires knowledge of managerial principles, how to apply them, and the ability to motivate, to challenge, and to inspire others to achieve success. It can be said that the ultimate example of leadership is soldiers in combat. Certainly, they must raise the question to themselves, "If we had a choice, would we want to follow our team leader into battle?" The program administrator must provide the evidence that the effort and energy utilized by the staff will make the difference.

MANAGERIAL PRACTICES

Sullivant and Decker (1988) remind us that one common problem that has been found in many bureaucratic organizations, especially those without clear-cut goals, is *goal displacement. Goal displacement means that a department pursues its own narrowly defined goals rather than the overall goals of the institution.* It is not only important for an institution to establish objectives, but each individual in the institution should be involved in the process.

Deegan (1977) describes one technique for doing this, which has become known as *"management by objective"* (MBO). Such an approach has several stages. The first stage is the determination of the overall objectives of the institution set by top management. These objectives are shared with department heads, who then formulate objectives for their particular work units. These latter objectives are discussed by the department heads and their subordinates to ensure that health care organization and departmental objectives are compatible. Deegan points out that once the objectives are formulated, the subordinate works on developing a game plan to achieve them. Measures of achievement are predetermined, and feedback as to whether, or to what degree, the objectives are achieved is given to the subordinate at specified intervals (Figure 1–1).

The concept of MBO to set operating goals probably has frustrated more leaders and managers than any other technique (Ross, 1986, Walton, 1986). According to Ross (1986):

> The weakness in implementing an MBO process surfaces in the second or third levels of an organization. Too frequently, these managers are poorly equipped to set measurable goals, since tradition dictates that goal setting starts only at the top. To further complicate the picture, the competency of first-line supervisors varies immensely. (p. 22)

Deegan (1977) tells us MBO is most effective in work environments where there are clear-cut institutional objectives. He points out that top executives in the hierarchy of the organization actively recruit lower-level participation in departmental goal setting and in measuring individual outcomes. Feedback is ongoing to ensure considerable trust and motivation between the department manager, supervisors, and their subordinates. Deegan concludes that some would argue that the above situation represents a very favorable work environment and that MBO is likely to work best where it is needed the least. Nevertheless, the setting of objectives is an important administrative function.

Sholtes (1988), in discussing top management's criticism of MBO, tells us it is a system of numerical objectives, standards, and quotas which does not emphasize processes and systems, and rewarded efforts are short term. Health care management experts often ask, "Is there a better alternative?" The alternative process, we believe, is the Deming Management Method (Walton, 1986). It is also referred to as *total quality management* (TQM), *continuous quality improvement* (CQI), or *quality improvement* (QI). In any case, *QI emphasizes results by working on methods. It entails a never-satisfied attitude, which supports an ongoing process to improve clinical and service outcomes.* Problems are solved, not just covered up. Scholtes (1988) reminds us that the client's concerns are given top priority to evaluate and constantly improve upon, so that the final product or service exceeds client expectations. Without a doubt, this can only be achieved by building excellence into every aspect of the work environment. QI, therefore, focuses on creating a work environment that encourages everyone to contribute to the company. Everyone in the organization learns to solve problems and make improvements (Walton, 1986). Each process is carefully described, problems identified, and the causes of problems determined through careful study. Then new error-proof methods are developed. Every process is brought under statistical control. Variation is studied, understood, and reduced well beyond specifications, and then it is reduced even more. As improvement occurs, processes are executed more successfully. *Productivity goes up as waste and inefficiency go down.* Clients receive products and services of higher value at lower costs. The significance is that anyone who receives better quality and low cost will tell others, and the demand for the product or service will increase. The proponent of QI is W. Edwards Deming, PhD and his methodology has become known as the Deming Chain Reaction (Figure 1–2). For a more comprehensive treatment on the topic of Quality Improvement, the reader is referred to Chapter 5.

Individuals exposed to only one management model initially may base their management style on what they have learned in the past. Those with a wider base of experience may approach leadership issues differently, through the use of a variety of solutions to address specific problems. The extent of leadership used by department managers indicates much about their perception of trust.

THE INFLUENCE OF THE ASLP ADMINISTRATOR

Change presents both challenges and opportunities, and there is a call for leadership from ASLP administrators. The traditional view of administration was that it existed to ensure that systems, processes, equipment, and other essential tools, were in place to support the provision of communication health care as determined by physicians and clients. However, we can no longer concentrate primarily on resource management skills. We must direct our attention to quality of care, the delivery of products and services, and the ways in which we can encourage change. ASLP administrators must be both leaders and managers in their departments. Bennis and Nanus (1985, p. 20) wrote, "Leadership is what gives an organization its vision and its ability to translate that vision into reality." They defined management as "to bring about, to have charge of or responsibility for, to conduct" and leadership as "influencing, guiding, in direction, course action, and opinion."

Administrators must adopt a departmental vision that is consistent with the views and management style of the entire organization. We must lead our departments by focusing on mission, direction, and role— in other words, the vision of the department. Therefore, the emphasis is on planning, and effective planning requires the skills of both leaders

A. GOALS

    Healthcare Organization

    1. Effectively develop services to be offered by the medical center.
    2. Manage financial and human resources in a manner which demonstrates commitment to cost effectiveness, improved productivity, and quality service.

    ASLP Department

    1. Effectively develop ASLP services to be offered by the department.
    2. Manage ALSP resources in a similar manner.

B. OBJECTIVES:

    Healthcare Organization:

    1. Prepare plans for developing services.
    2. Establish unilateral cost containment programs for each department.

    ASLP Department:

    1. Prepare and submit plans for developing ASLP.
    2. Establish unilateral cost containment programs for each department.

C. DATE OF COMPLETION:

    Healthcare Organization

    1. June 1, 1993
    2. June 1, 1993

    ASLP Department

    1. June 1, 1993
    2. June 1, 1993

(continued)

Figure 1–1. Management by Objectives process used to determine if the objectives of the health care organization and the ASLP department have been achieved.

and managers. Administrators must lead the way and not just respond to environmental factors. Proactive administrators need to decide what has to happen, and then make it happen. Cole, Benfer, Darrity, and Bellware (1991) list five attributes of proactive administrators:

■ Strategic thinking.
■ Leadership. Too many organizations are overmanaged and underled.
■ Enpowerment. An organization that has committed people can achieve almost anything.

(continued)

D. WEIGHT (%)

Healthcare Organization

1. 100%
   0%
2. 100%
   0%

ASLP Department

1. 100%
   0%
2. 100%
   0%

E. DEFINITION OF SUCCESS OR FAILURE:

Healthcare Organization

1. Success: Study submitted to CEO on time.
   Failure: Study not completed.
2. Success: Study submitted to CEO on time.
   Failure: Study not completed.

ASLP Department

1. Success: Study submitted to CEO on time.
   Failure: Study not completed.
2. Success: Study submitted to CEO on time.
   Failure: Study not completed.

■ Risk-taker. The reallocation of financial dollars (put the money where the work is) within a department or competing against similar programs involves risk.

■ Process-oriented. Proactive administrators require building long-term operational processes and systems.

In addition, administrators will be involved in program development, financial management, developing quality monitoring systems, human resource management, maintaining productivity, and the marketing of clinical services. The challenges that we administrators face to influence and successfully direct a change in ASLP policies require professionals who can not only conceptualize and understand cause and

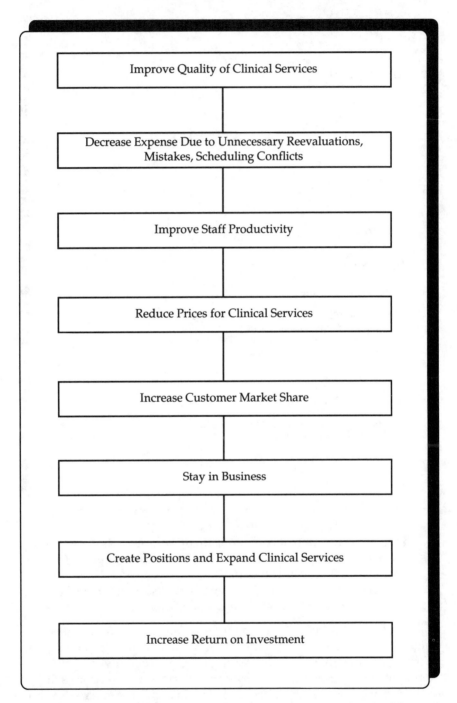

Figure 1–2. The Deming Chain Reaction improvement process applied to the delivery of ASLP health care services.

effect relationships, but can also create the strategic actions needed to effect the outcome they desire. These people are referred to as ASLP leaders.

MANAGERIAL FUNCTIONS

Haimann (1989) classifies managerial function into five primary categories: planning, organizing, staffing, influencing, and controlling.

Planning

Planning for service excellence needs to be meticulous, comprehensive, and thoughtful. *Planning entails determining what should be done, and why, where, by whom, when, and how it should be done.* The goal of planning is to ensure that the objectives, policies, procedures, methods, rules, budgets, and other plans are carefully adapted to fit the department's current realities and its problems, culture, and staff. Department managers must determine in advance the goals to be achieved, the direction to take, and the best means to achieve these objectives.

Deane (1990), in discussing planning, tells us that this first managerial function can be separated into three categories:

■ Directional planning involves determining the mission, overall direction, departmental role, and clarification of values pertaining to management and the provision of services.

■ Strategic planning involves establishing priorities, developing programs/services, and determining the geographic area that will be served.

■ Operational planning involves establishing and implementing plans related to programs, technology, facilities, human resources, finances, information systems, quality assurance, and so forth.

An important part of the operational plan is to create a *competitive advantage* for the ASLP department in the market place. To achieve this, department managers should answer the following questions on competitive position, image, organizational culture, administration, staff, and health care professionals:

■ How is the ASLP department doing financially? Is patient activity up or down? What are the trends?

■ Are there any financial problems? What is the status of the profit-and-loss statement (to be discussed in Chapter 8)?

■ Are there any population(s) and economic trends that face the department? What is the economy in the local area? How does this affect the reimbursement?

■ Who is the competition?

- What is the public's perception of the ASLP department? What kind of reputation does the department really have?
- How do other professionals perceive the department? How do patients rate the quality of service?
- Are there any complaints about the quality of service?
- What is the culture of the health care organization? Of the department? Is it friendly, open, caring, impersonal, cold, unfriendly?
- What are the employees' views toward one another, top management, toward physicians, supervisors, and their positions?
- Have any new programs been initiated? Are employees involved in decision-making?
- What standards of behavior do staff members use in client relations? Is the staff consumer-oriented?
- Does the staff resist change?
- Do members of the staff trust one another? Why? Why not?
- How does the staff feel about the work environment? Is there considerable staff turnover? If so, why? Is productivity high or low?
- Does the administrator "manage by walking around"?
- Does the administrator communicate with the staff? If so, how often?
- How often does the administrator meet with supervisors to keep them informed of managerial issues?
- Does the administrator circulate a monthly information bulletin of upcoming events and accomplishments?
- Does the staff take pride in their work, their appearance?
- How much cooperation exists between the staff and other health care professionals?

Information that is truly useful in planning must take into consideration the objectives of the organization, as set forth by the *chief executive officer* (CEO), conversations with top management, employees, other professionals' opinions, and patient surveys. Sullivant and Decker (1988) point out that planning must come before any of the other managerial functions. From these initial plans then come specific policies to achieve departmental and organizational goals. Procedures, rules and regulations, schedules, and budgets are established as part of the overall departmental plan. Sullivant and Decker conclude that the function of planning continues in revising the course of action and choosing different alternatives as the need arises.

Organizing

Organizing refers to the structure within which things get done, and determines how to align available resources to serve the organization's purpose. Once a strategic plan has been developed, the department managers' organizational skills will determine how the work is to be accomplished. They must define, group, and assign job responsibilities and tasks that are evenly distributed to various groups, divisions, sections, teams, or other work units. In other words, to organize means to assign fixed responsibilities to departmental specialty units and individuals who work for the department, to assign particular duties to these positions, and to delegate a certain amount of authority to the subordinate supervisors, so that they can carry out the duties for which they are responsible. To achieve results from organizing the department, the ASLP administrator should ask the following questions:

■ Does the department have written objectives?
■ Does the entire staff support departmental objectives?
■ Do all staff members participate in the establishment of objectives?
■ Are members of the staff held accountable for writing and meeting objectives?
■ Are all position descriptions (to be discussed in Chapter 4) current?
■ Are the lines of communication clearly defined in the organizational chart?
■ Are all members of the staff kept informed of organizational changes that affect their functions?
■ Are departmental policies available for the staff to review and do members of the staff know their responsibilities in carrying out these policies?
■ Is there a plan for development, review, and approval of departmental procedures?
■ Are the procedure manuals current?
■ Does the administrative staff have an appropriate understanding of the department's functions?

The organizing process will result in the creation of an activity-authority network for the ASLP department, which is a subsystem within the total health care network. For a more in-depth discussion on the topic of organizing ASLP health care programs, the reader is referred to Chapter 2.

Staffing

The ASLP administrator is responsible for recruiting and selecting qualified employees to fill the various positions in the department. In recent years, the concept of professional standards and quality assurance have prompted changes in the focus of clinical practice, from simply filling staff positions to developing integrated health care. ASLP administrators are challenged to set high standards of practice by establishing continuing education programs for staff development, promoting them, appraising their performance, and giving them opportunities for further improvement. In addition, staffing includes a justifiable system of compensation. In most health care organizations, the *human resource management* (HRM) department provides the technical support to assist in various aspects of staffing. However, formal authority and responsibility for staff recruitment remains with the ASLP administrator. For a more comprehensive treatment on the topic of HRM, the reader is referred to Chapter 4.

Influencing

Haimann (1989) informs us that influencing is assigning specific resources to accomplish specific tasks as required. In simple terms, *influencing involves running the organization on a daily basis.* This means giving notification to staff members on how to accomplish their jobs and helping them work together. He adds that influencing is a process that includes "guiding, teaching, coaching, and supervising subordinates" (p. 15). Hence, the adage, "I will lead if you will follow," and if no one leads, no one follows. Haimann tells us that the administrator must "motivate the staff to achieve their maximum potential, satisfy their needs, and stimulate them to act in ways they may not on their own" (p. 15).

Therefore, influencing is a process that entails studying the desires of the employees, morale, job satisfaction, productivity, leadership, and communication. Influencing affords the administrator the opportunity to create an atmosphere that will enhance employee motivation while focusing on the goals and objectives of the health care organization.

Controlling

Controlling consists of integrating activities and balancing tasks so that appropriate actions take place in the proper place and time. The most important aspect of controlling is authority. Without authority a person in an organizational setting cannot be a leader. According to Webster's *Ninth New Collegiate Dictionary*, authority is defined as: (1) a power to influence or command thought, opinion, or behavior; (2) persons in command; and, (3) a convincing force. Haimann points out that power represents the byproduct by which the subordinates perform or do not perform a specific assignment. In discussing power, he tells us the administrator can, to a certain extent, control the actions of the employee. Most often, top management empowers department heads to oversee their work units and make all decisions with regard to the work of that group. As a leader, the program administrator must take the responsibility for attaining an objective. Once an individual assumes the leadership of a group, that person alone is responsible for reaching the objective. Haimann further states that managerial authority is not assigned to people but to the formal title of the position within the organization.

The possession of power must also include the authority to impose limitations, when necessary. For example, if a subordinate refuses to carry out a certain assignment, this authority must include the right to take disciplinary action, and possibly to recommend dismissal of the employee. Haimann notes that this aspect of authority obviously has many limitations in the form of legal restrictions, union contracts, or consideration of morals, ethics, and human behavior. For example, legal restrictions require that an appropriate process be followed prior to dismissing an employee. He reminds us that successful administrators should not depend on formal authority, but should use other mechanisms to encourage subordinates to accomplish the job. In other words, think positively and do not dwell on the negative aspects of authority. Today, proactive administrators use terms such as responsibility, tasks, or duties, instead of the term authority. The emphasis should be on having the responsibility for certain activities instead of saying that they possess authority. A great administrator is an influential manager of people and resources who accepts responsibility for himself, his actions, and any results.

Control is the function that looks at what actually happened and makes adjustments to encourage the outcome to conform with expected or required results. In other words, *to control means to establish the plans to be carried out, to monitor what progress is being made toward the objectives, and to determine whether other corrective actions must be taken to remedy all deviations.* Managerial practices (e.g., MBO, TQM, CQI, or QI), previously mentioned, can also be considered as control mechanisms.

The program administrator should view these five managerial functions as a continuous cycle of activity that affects the outcome of each other.

EFFECTIVE COMMUNICATION

There is a direct relationship between effective management and effective communication. Fulmer (1983) and Ziglar (1986) point out some key elements to remember in communicating with others:

- Clarity. Communication should be to the point and easily understood.
- Completeness. Part of the message is sometimes more harmful than no message at all.
- Conciseness. The speaker must clearly describe the specific message to be conveyed, choosing words properly, and avoiding verbosity. Words should be selected that comprise the listener's (not the sender's) level of experience.
- Concreteness. Speakers usually revert to abstract or generalized statements when they are unable to provide the facts.
- Correctness. Communication is ineffective if the message is incorrect or not sincere.
- Timing. Good communication presented at the wrong time is considered poor communication.
- Feedback. Make adjustments on future actions based upon information about past performance.

- ■ Credibility. Being trustworthy, reliable, and competent are characteristics of a credible professional. Remember the rule, "Say what you mean and mean what you say."
- ■ Recognition. The employment atmosphere should acknowledge the individual contributions of others and should be viewed as complimentary in nature. Remember, praise in public and criticize in private.

Department managers who devote sufficient time to these areas will substantially increase the effectiveness of their communication skills.

Downward Communication

Downward communication (e.g., between the administrator and a subordinate) implies specific instructions for the subordinate. This method allows the administrator to integrate personnel management activities and to use human resources more effectively. The department manager may be responsible for staff recruitment, conducting interviews/counseling sessions, disciplining employees, handling complaints, and settling differences. Effective communication is a prerequisite to building and maintaining an effective working relationship. Ziglar (1986) lists some excellent guidelines for developing a successful message strategy:

- ■ Listen and communicate.
- ■ Communicate understanding and recognition.
- ■ Communicate participative management.
- ■ Communicate initiatives through "parenting."
- ■ Communicate trust, mission, and expectations.
- ■ Communicate confidence.
- ■ Communicate fun and happiness.
- ■ Communicate expectations.

The department manager is responsible both for quality of patient care and for the quality of work life of each staff member. It is essential that a balance between these two sets of needs be pursued.

Upward Communication with Superiors

The department manager's ability to communicate with top management can be compared to the communication that exists between the program administrator and subordinates; however, the administrator is now the subordinate. Nevertheless, the principles and practices used in communicating with subordinates are equally appropriate in this situation. ASLP administrators must develop responsible communication concerning departmental decisions for initiating requests, in public relations, and in future issues that may affect the health care organizations. They must also be prepared to listen objectively to the comments made by their superiors and be willing to consider alternative measures, in order to avoid "turf disputes" with other departments.

Communication With The Medical Staff

Communication with the medical staff can be a challenge for clinical department managers because of the nature of the relationship between physicians and allied health professionals and because of the gender disparity within both professions (with a great preponderance of male physicians and female ASLPs). Wilford (1986) points out that anyone presenting new ideas to physicians should be prepared to repeat themselves several times. He states the response to the initial presentation is usually negative, the second presentation generates some understanding, and after the third presentation, if it is desirable, the department manager should expect acceptance. Wilford concludes that patience is a special quality to have when communicating with physicians. He advises us to communicate with physicians informally (e.g., in their offices) to resolve differences of opinion and to prevent the risk of embarrassment.

Communication with Other Health Care Professionals

Horizontal and lateral communication refers to communication between people on the same level with comparable authority. Coordination of activities and planning are enhanced through effective communication among staff members within a department or between various departments within the health care organization. The ASLP administrator must utilize considerable tact in communicating with personnel and other department managers. Here, the ASLP administrator must recognize and respond to the differences between the goals of their departments and other units in order to create an environment for commonality of purpose.

Written Communication

Most written communication in management is formal and includes such tasks as:

■ Preparing job descriptions, performance appraisals, or reports of contact;

■ Preparing documents of activity, financial reports, justification for new equipment, additional space, and staff;

■ Recording committee activities, including agenda and minutes; and,

■ Developing written policies and procedures for the department.

The preparation of job descriptions and employee performance appraisals is a difficult and disliked management responsibility, yet an integral part of managerial practice. In recent years, concepts involving job descriptions have enabled an institution to focus on ASLP practice, from simple job descriptions to integrated systems. Job descriptions delineate appropriate tasks to be performed that are consistent with the department's needs. Department managers are challenged to write accurate job descriptions in order to integrate clinical practice into standards of performance evaluation. This will reduce the influence of personality factors, and focuses the appraisal on the tasks performed and the quality of the performance. Written communication and the face-to-face appraisal interview are usually more effective in specifying areas of strength or weaknesses in need of improvement. Effective written and oral communication skills are essential in carrying out this responsibility. For a more in-depth discussion on the topic of human resource management (HRM), see Chapter 4.

Listening

Active listening plays an essential role in the administrator-subordinate relationship. This means paying attention to the speaker, including body language, eye contact, vocabulary, and voice volume. Department managers must ensure that all communication is within the subordinate's level of comprehension (e.g., past experiences, attitudes, biases, and preconceptions).

Metzger (1988) offers some points to consider to assist in developing active listening skills:

■ Maintain direct face-to-face contact.
■ Keep an open posture.
■ Lean toward the other person.
■ Maintain good eye contact.
■ Be relaxed.
■ Display attentiveness through facial expression.
■ Attend with vocal cues.

Effective communication skills are essential tools for the ASLP administrator to use in managing the department. These skills, like many others, can be learned. Communication is an interactive process that occurs between a sender and a receiver. It includes oral, verbal, nonverbal, and written communication. Principles of effective communication include accepting responsibility for sending a clear message, using appropriate language, and encouraging feedback.

MEETINGS

A meeting refers to a group of people who have come together for a common purpose. The challenge of the department manager is to ensure that the purpose is accomplished. In clinical practice, meetings are frequent and are an essential part of doing business. Gee and Teig (1986) remind us that meetings are held to disseminate information, develop policies and procedures, enforce regulations and legal requirements, instill confidence, perform technical functions, develop plans and strategies, and to make decisions. They tell us, "The choice of subject matter, participants, location, date and time, meeting logistics, and meeting strategies all become crucial to successful outcomes" (p. 103).

The Health Care Education Associates (HCEA) (1987) identify four different types of committees:

∎ Standing Committee. This committee meets on a regular basis and is comprised of members from different positions or groups within an organization who discuss, in general, quality assurance standards, continuing education, and equipment-related issues.

∎ Steering Committee. This committee also meets on a regular basis and is composed of members from the same department who discuss operational issues (e.g., staff development and supervisory or administrative issues).

∎ Task Force Committee. This type of committee is established on a temporary basis, the intent being that once the particular mission (task) is fulfilled (e.g., special events, search committee, specific situations, or problems), the committee is abolished. Nowadays, this committee may be referred to as a process action team (to be discussed in Chapter 5).

∎ Interdepartmental Committee. This type of committee is composed of members who represent different departments in the health care organization (e.g., ASLP, Otolaryngology, Neurology, Nursing, etc.) who attempt to identify and improve departmental concerns.

Whatever name is applied, the goal(s) and objective(s) of the committee need(s) to be established clearly since it is difficult for a meeting group to deal with abstract concepts. Meeting objectives should support the general goals of a committee. Goals usually have a long-term time frame and refer to the overall purpose of the committee. On the other hand, objectives usually have a shorter time frame and refer to the purpose of specific meetings. HCEA (1987) points out that meeting objectives should support the general goals of a committee, for example:

∎ To disseminate information (e.g., to provide the committee with a status report of what is happening in another area).

∎ To identify a need, solve a problem, improve the quality of care or services, seek different points of view, or to discuss topics concerning future program direction.

∎ To develop quality assurance standards.

∎ To assign action responsibilities or to identify and plan details for a program or activity (e.g., plan an activity).

- To interview and evaluate candidates for positions.
- To make recommendations for purchase of equipment and supplies, to identify new market shares, to develop strategies for the delivery of services.

Prior to the meeting, the preparation of the agenda is the responsibility of the chairperson and the secretary. The agenda items should be prioritized. We recommend that quality assurance and quality control activities be the first agenda items for staff meetings in all clinical departments. Each topic (aspect of care) should be separated as a unique item for discussion. The format for preparing meeting minutes can follow the example shown in Figure 1–3. It is important for the committee chairperson to specify the amount of time allotted to the subject matter so that a schedule can be maintained. This may not be a requirement if the chairperson is in control of the committee.

Room reservations and any special arrangements (e.g., audiovisual equipment, etc.) should be made in advance. This will prevent chaos that may result when meeting rooms are found to be occupied by staff from other departments or because of equipment breakdown. Meetings that begin effortlessly will allow the committee to achieve its desired outcome. Otherwise, everyone has wasted time, and time is money.

Recurring meetings should be scheduled a year in advance to ensure that attendees will make adjustments to their schedules. Committee members who are expected to review complex issues should be provided with background material no later than four or five days beforehand so that the participants have adequate time to evaluate the material.

Meeting Minutes

HCEA (1987) tells us that that meeting minutes (which serve as an official document of activities that were discussed during the previous meeting) are required by regulatory agencies. Minutes allow department members to determine if the objectives of the committee are being met. HCEA points out that meeting minutes also provide a source of continuity. Committee members can read the minutes of previous meetings to refresh their minds about events that have been previously discussed. The minutes reflect the actions of a specific group of people for a specific time frame.

The secretary is responsible for generating minutes of the meeting. Minutes can be extremely short (one-page summary) to lengthy transcripts. Gee and Teig (1986) suggest that minutes capture the essence of the discussion and outcome without having to duplicate every detail. Minutes should contain the name of the department, the date/time, place of the meeting, attendees, the body of the minutes, with action requirements either underlined or otherwise highlighted for easy identification, the time the committee adjourned, and the signature of the

Anywhere Medical Center

_____ Chief of Staff
_____ QA Coordinator

Audiology-Speech-Language Pathology
Monthly Staff Meeting Minutes

DATE:

Convened:
Adjourned:

Present:
   Late:
Absent:

A. Quality Improvement:

   Dr. Smith discussed with the staff the QA monitors for the month of June, 1993.

   (1) Aspect(s) of Care: Hearing Aid Management, Dysphagia Management, and so
                                   forth.

       Findings: Results of the Audit.

       Conclusions: Analysis of the data, identification of trends or
                                   patterns.

       Recommendations: Desired improvement based on the conclusions.

       Actions: What is to be implemented based on recommendations,
                                   stating who, when, how, and date to be completed.

       Follow-up: Isolated deficiencies receive appropriate feedback as part
                                   of QI. System's problems require a change in policy or
                                   procedure to determine effective improvement.

B. New Policies and information:

C. Activities Report:

D. Safety, Occupational, Health, Fire Protection Report:

E. Other Topics Discussed:

Signature   Signature
Department Head   Secretary

Figure 1–3. Standardized staff meeting minutes. This format is used for the discussion of quality improvement and quality control. The use of this format for other agenda is optional.

chairman and secretary. The secretary should provide attendees with the minutes in hours (e.g., within 24 hours, 48 hours maximum). Nothing is more frustrating than to receive minutes for a meeting you can barely remember.

HCEA (1987) offers some useful checkpoints for recording of meeting minutes:

- Minutes should be double-spaced to facilitate corrections.
- Agenda items, or topics, should be numbered consecutively for quick reference.
- Each page of official minutes should be numbered consecutively and should be kept in a loose-leaf binder.
- The language should be clear, and abbreviations should be avoided.
- Any corrections to the minutes of a previous meeting should be approved by the committee. The recording secretary should draw a red line through the words or paragraph to be deleted, with the appropriate substitution written directly above or on another sheet of paper entitled "Addendum."
- When referring to individual persons by name, use complete names or titles.
- Recording of the discussion should be kept to a minimum. Only relevant information that relates to the topic should be recorded.
- Retain the original copy of minutes in department files.
- Committee members, both present or absent, should receive a copy of the minutes.

As a further note, the chairpersons should determine the effectiveness of their meetings by asking committee members the following questions: First, how well is the committee functioning under their leadership? Second, are the objectives of the meeting being met? Do all committee members contribute equally, or is the meeting comprised of people that talk and those that don't? Three, are there any problems? Is there a plan for dealing with these problems?

This evaluation increases self-awareness among committee members. Standing committees, as mandated by regulatory bodies or the health care organizations bylaws, will need members, a chairperson, and secretary. The chairperson has the responsibility of starting the meeting on time, steering the meeting along the agenda track, assigning responsibilities, and adjourning on time when its mission has been fulfilled. Gee and Teig (1986) advise us that meetings should have a maximum time obligation (e.g., one hour). They tell us that a chairperson should start the meeting on time, even if key staff are not present. This approach will let the staff know who is in charge.

In this era of QI, meetings must be outcome-oriented. However, some meetings require adherence to formalized protocol, especially if there is wide divergency in viewpoints. There are rulebooks that exist governing meeting conduct (e.g., *Robert's Rules of Order*). However, department heads seeking staff participation and agreement are likely to avoid such formalities. Nevertheless, it is beneficial to read such a rulebook since it tends to organize the sequences of a meeting in an orderly fashion.

MOTIVATION

The general trend in health care in recent years has been toward growing employee dissatisfaction. Complaints have less to do with money and more to do with the work environment. The problem is not in the work, rather the problem lies in those who create and control the work environment. Motivation of employees is of great importance to administrators because of its impact on performance. Motivation is closely related to the managerial function of influencing (previously discussed), because it deals directly with the individual. The only true motivation is internal, which can be sustained and controlled. Contemporary administrators must understand that the old "do-it-or-else" style of motivation is obsolete. Understanding motivation will enable managers to help their employees achieve higher levels of job satisfaction and job performance.

Most management books often cite the behavioral sciences' view of motivation; however this can be so boring and difficult to understand. Our approach will be to adapt contemporary theories (e.g., Maslow, 1943; McGregor, 1960; Ouichi, 1981), most often discussed, to the work environment.

Abraham H. Maslow's model contains five levels of human need, for example:

■ Physiological needs are met in the work environment by providing adequate wages to enable an individual to obtain the necessities and comforts of life.

■ Safety needs are met in the work environment through job security, favorable management action, no justifiable complaints of discrimination, predictable administration, and so forth.

■ Social needs consist of a sense of belonging to the organization, acceptance by one's peers, and giving and receiving respect and understanding.

■ Self-esteem focuses on one's desire to have a worthy self-image and to receive recognition from others. These needs for esteem involve both self-esteem and esteem from others. These needs are often fulfilled by mastery over subject matter, for example, by knowing that you can accomplish a certain task.

■ Self-actualization or self-fulfillment is the need for realizing one's own potential, for continued self-development, or for being creative. In other words, this is the need to maximize one's abilities. Unlike the other four needs, which probably will result in personal satisfaction, self-actualization is seldom fully achieved. Since this need is probably internalized, the ASLP administrator should strive to create an environment conducive to self-actualization.

Conditions of modern life give many people little opportunity to fulfill the need for self-actualization. Most employees are continuously struggling to satisfy their lower needs, investing most of their energy to satisfy them. Therefore, the need for self-fulfillment frequently remains dormant and unfulfilled. Self-actualization is often the basis of conflict between organizational and individual goals.

In 1960, Douglas McGregor (author of *The Human Side Of Enterprise*) developed two opposing views of workers' attitudes based upon different concepts of management styles. Theory X represented bureaucratic and authoritarian attitudes toward employees. Its basic assumption was that people are inherently lazy, do not like to work, and can only be motivated or coerced by external rewards, and people prefer close supervision. In contrast, Theory Y represented a democratic approach, which provides the employee with the opportunity for creativity and responsibility. Its basic assumption was that people were highly motivated and liked to work, had an inherent drive for growth, development, and self-actualization, and wanted to share in the decision making.

Theory Z is a term coined by W.G. Ouichi (1981) to describe the Japanese style of management. He used the term in contrast with Theory X and Theory Y. The basic assumption of Theory Z is that involved workers are the key to productivity, and everything else is secondary. It recognizes that people are composed of both Theories X and Y, and that the challenge lies in creating a common culture in which the organization realizes it can meet the objectives of the people. Involvement is brought about through the development of trust, subtlety, and intimacy. In 1986, Zig Ziglar in his book *Top Performance* said, "people don't care how much you know, until they know how much you care . . . about them" (p. 110).

If department managers really want motivated employees, they should use stimulators such as achievement, recognition, the work itself, responsibility, and advancement. These are the factors that, if present, truly stimulate people. Opportunities for career advancement, greater responsibility, the possibility of promotion, growth, achievement, and interesting work make any position challenging, meaningful, and really motivate subordinates. Such stimulators are obviously associated with the previously discussed higher-order needs of people. The essence of good management is letting the staff know your expectations, inspecting what is done, and rewarding those things that are done well. Once department managers identify the behavior that constitutes excellence, they should establish a formal reward and recognition program. Ziglar (1986) offers us some checkpoints to assist us:

- Recognize things that are important to the employees.
- Employees must buy into the reward and recognition program, assured that it is administered fairly.
- Control the "brown nosing" behaviors present in the department. Establish awards for individual heroic acts, others for consistent daily performance, and some for team effort that exemplifies the behavior you expect.
- Establish objective standards for rewarding staff.
- Recognize winners regularly and promptly (e.g., at monthly departmental meetings, a note from top management, monetary award, or a commendation). The best reward is still an immediate acknowledgment from the supervisor.
- Reward improvement, not just excellence. Neophyte clinicians need time to refine and smooth out their skills, even though they received academic training and are continuing to work toward improvement. Encourage them.
- Do not recognize inferior performance. If there are no winners in a particular category, it is better to say so than to award someone who is undeserving.

CONFLICTS BETWEEN INDIVIDUAL AND DEPARTMENTAL GOALS

The primary cause of conflict exists when individual needs and goals conflict rather than coincide with those of the department. Haimann (1989) tells us that numerous reports exist on the topic concerning individuals who want to be stimulated and independent, and work in a large bureaucratic organization. This issue has severe consequences that can result in high turnover, lower productivity, lethargic behavior, lack of innovation and creativity, non-approval of leadership, and so forth. ASLP administrators who work in large health care settings are becoming more aware of these consequences and of the necessity for an organization to provide a climate that will motivate its employees toward personal satisfaction. Ziglar (1986) and Cohen (1990) make some cogent recommendations to achieve a healthy work environment:

- Show respect for a job well done.
- Involve employees in decision making.
- Be short on promises and long on fulfillment.
- Keep an open mind.
- Respect the opinions and feelings of others.
- Communicate effectively.
- Make sure the employees know what is to be expected.
- Prevent boredom and low morale.

■ Make the job more interesting.
■ Have clearly defined goals and objectives.
■ Be human, don't fear to make a mistake.
■ Encourage self-discipline and self-esteem.

Since employee morale is affected by many factors, in and outside the work place, those who have confidence in management's integrity are most likely to deliver their best work and to do so consistently. The best way management can build this confidence in itself is to communicate its abilities honestly, confidently, and directly. After all, a well run department will help build the best employee morale.

STRESS MANAGEMENT

Steers (1984) defines stress as "the reaction of individuals to demands from the environment that pose a threat" (p. 506). What are those forces in health care that have created stress-induced diseases? In addition to the stress imposed by society and family, ASLP administrators face additional stress because of the idiosyncrasies associated with the profession. For example, the delivery of services, interactions among staff members who form the power base of the department within the health care organization, the influence of outside regulatory groups including third-party payers, the threat of malpractice, and more. ASLP administrators also worry about keeping abreast of contemporary knowledge, state-of-the-art technology, new delivery systems/markets, reorganizational needs, reimbursement strategies, government regulation, and so on.

As a result, burnout can have a devastating effect not only on the careers, health, and happiness of department managers but also on the organization they represent. Enthusiasm and effectiveness can be lost or subdued, creating a chain reaction that may affect all employees in the department. Burned-out administrators do not have the initiative to pursue higher career goals, motivate employees, promote company growth, or effectively manage the department's daily activities.

The question to ask, then, is "If being a department manager is so stressful, why does anyone assume these positions?" The answer is obvious: There are effective ways to adapt and cope with stress. No doubt, the complexities inherent in ASLP will continue to intensify, particularly in the era of cost containment versus quality of care. The effective formula for avoiding the burnout route is quite simple: *exercise*. Running is an excellent choice. While this form of activity may not be welcomed by many, the important thing is that you keep your heartbeat up for at least 20 minutes approximately four times per week (Galloway, 1984). Fast walking, aerobics, riding a stationary bike, racquetball, handball, rowing, using step climbers, cross-country ski machines, and swimming are all excellent forms of exercise. Exercise activates the pituitary gland which floods the body with endorphines, which are more than two hundred times more powerful than morphine. The benefit to the individual is a "natural chemical high" for two to as much four or five hours. An hour invested at noon (counting time to undress, exercise, shower, cool down, etc.) returns two-to-four times that much high productivity time. Hence, the effective work day is extended by several hours. A narrative that best describes the benefits of working out regularly is entitled:

WHAT IS A WORKOUT?

A workout is 25 per cent perspiration and 75 per cent determination. Stated another way, it is one-part physical exertion and three parts self-discipline. Doing it is easy once you get started.

A workout makes you better today than you were yesterday. It strengthens the body, relaxes the mind, and toughens the spirit. When you work out regularly, your problems diminish and your confidence grows.

A workout is a personal triumph over laziness and procrastination. It is the badge of a winner, the mark of an organized, goal-oriented person who has taken charge of his or her destiny.

A workout is a wise investment of time and an investment in excellence. It is a way of preparing for life's challenges and proving to yourself that you have what it takes to do what is necessary.

A workout is a key that helps unlock the door to opportunity and success. Hidden within each of us is an extraordinary force. Physical and mental fitness are the triggers that can release it.

A workout is a form of rebirth. When you finish a good workout, you don't simply feel better,

YOU FEEL BETTER ABOUT YOURSELF.

This natural reward will sustain the individual who can stick with an exercise program for six months. It may not even take that long, but if it does, six months is not a big investment for improved health, fitness, and performance for the rest of your life. Before beginning any exercise program, it is advisable to get a thorough physical examination. Information on blood pressure, cholesterol level, resting pulse rate, breathing rate, weight, and measurements will serve as a reference point for measuring fitness improvement.

In addition to exercise, a well-balanced diet should be maintained, with sufficient amounts of carbohydrates (e.g., Four Food Group Plan—dairy, protein, fruit/vegetable, and grain). A sensible diet rich in carbohydrates not only provides adequate muscle glycogen storage that sustains the individual through the course of the day, but also helps prevent heart disease, stroke, and cancer (Coleman, 1988). In the words of William Shakespeare, "Our bodies are our gardens, our wills are gardeners."

CONCLUSION

It can be said that leadership is an exercise in which not one individual has exclusive authority, but in which relatively many are involved. Certainly, in our profession we are dependent on leaders at every level of our organizational structure (i.e., local, state, and national). Leadership in the ASLP profession is dispersed to an extraordinary degree. Every ASLP has the potential of exerting influence and is to that extent, a leader. At the same time, all of us have been, and will continue to be, influenced by others and so must, to a certain extent, be followers as well.

The public perception of ASLP is a composite of experiences involved in the individual clinician-patient relationship. Our public perception cannot and must not be taken for granted. We have been endowed with the heritage of those who came before us, and it is our responsibility to preserve this legacy for those who come after us. Indeed, leadership is a hollow word unless conditions are met to help ASLPs working at every level cope in their everyday professional and personal lives. Leadership is the frosting on the cake. In world politics, there are no world managers, just world leaders. Therefore, manage yourself, lead others.

To help develop more diverse leadership and management skills, we will deal in subsequent chapters with issues related to organizing ASLP programs, planning and designing facilities, human resource management, quality improvement, managing productivity, computerized information systems, financial management, and the marketing of services.

REFERENCES

Atchison, T. (1990). Turn around, leaders: Is anyone following? *Hospitals, 64,* 50–52.

Bennis, W., & Nanus, B. (1985). *Leaders: The strategies for taking charge.* Philadelphia: Harper & Row.

Cohen, W. A. (1990). *The art of the leader.* Englewood Cliffs, NJ: Prentice Hall.

Cole, G., Benfer, D., Darrity, J., & Bellware, G. (1991). Proactive executives: Prospering in tough times. *Hospitals, 65,* 22–27.

Coleman, E. (1988). *Eating for endurance.* Palo Alto, CA: Bull Publishing Company.

Deane, K. (1990). Executive management leads the way. *Dimensions in Health Services, 67,* 36–37.

Deegan, A. X., III. (1977). *Management by objectives for hospitals.* Rockville, MD: Aspen Systems Corporation.

Flarey, D. L. (1991). Redesigning management roles: The executive challenge. *Journal of Nursing Administration, 21,* 40–45.

Fiedler, F. E. (1967). *A theory of leadership effectiveness.* New York: McGraw-Hill Book Company.

Fulmer, R. M. (1983). *The new management.* New York: Macmillan.

Galloway, J. (1984). *Galloway's book on running.* Bolinas, CA: Shelter Publications, Inc.

Gee, D. A., & Teig, C. D. (1986). Effective meetings. In T. F. Moore & E. A. Simendinger (Eds.), *The effective health care executive: A guide to a winning management style* (pp. 99–110). Rockville, MD: Aspen Publishers Inc.

Haimann, T. (1989). *Supervisory management for healthcare organizations.* St. Louis, MO: The Catholic Health Association of the United States.

Health Care Education Associates Professional Advancement Series. (1987). *Group leadership skills for nurse managers.* St. Louis, MO: C.V. Mosby Company.

Hershey, P., & Blanchard, K. H. (1982). *Management of organizational behavior utilizing human resources* (4th ed.). Englewood Cliffs, NJ: Prentice-Hall.

Hickman, C. R., & Silva, M. A. (1985). *Creating excellence: Managing culture, strategy , and change in the new age.* Audio Cassette Tape Series. Chicago, IL: Nightingale-Conant Corporation.

Korman, A. K. (1966). Consideration, initiating structure, and organizational criteria—a review. *Personnel Psychology, 19,* 349–61.

Liekert, R. (1961). *New patterns of management.* New York: McGraw-Hill Book Company.

Maslow, A. H. (1943). Theory of human motivation. *Psychological Review, 50,* 370–396.

Mayo, E. (1933). *The human problems of an industrial civilization.* New York: MacMillan Company.

McGregor, D. (1960). *The human side of enterprise.* New York: McGraw-Hill Book Company.

Metzger, N. (1988). *The health care supervisor's handbook.* Rockville, MD: Aspen Publishers, Inc.

Ouichi, W. G. (1981). *Theory Z : How American business can meet the Japanese challenge.* Reading, MA: Addison-Wesley Publishing Co.

Peters, T. J. (1982). *In search of excellence.* New York: Harper and Row.

Peters, T. J. (1987). *Thriving in chaos.* New York: Harper & Row.

Rizzo, S. R., Gutnick, H. N., & Stein, D. W. (1992). Survey of audiology & speech-language pathology university training program: Preparation in administration. Unpublished manuscript.

Ross, A. (1986). Leadership vs. management: What's the difference. In T. F. Moore & E. A. Simendinger (Eds.) *The effective health care executive: A guide to a winning management style* (pp.15–28). Rockville, MD: Aspen Publishers, Inc.

Scholtes, P. R. (1988). *The team handbook: How to use teams to improve quality.* Madison, WI: Joiner Associates Inc.

Simmons, W. J., & Bixby, N .B. (1989). A model for leadership in administrative practice. *Mt. Sinai Journal of Medicine, 56,* 429–434.

Steers, R. M. (1984). *Introduction to organizational behavior.* Santa Monica, CA: Goodyear.

Sullivant, E. J., & Decker, P. J. (1988). *Effective management in nursing.* Menlo Park, CA: Addison-Wesley Publishing Company.

Tannebaum, R., & Schmidt, W. H. (1958). How to choose a leadership pattern. *Harvard Business Review, 36,* 95–102.

Taylor, F. W. (1911). *The principles of scientific management.* New York: Harper & Brothers.

Walton, M. (1986). *The Deming management method.* New York: Putnam Publishing Group.

Wilford, D. S. (1986). Effective communication. In T. F. Moore & E. A. Simendinger (Eds.) *The effective health care executive: A guide to a winning management style* (pp. 57–88). Rockville, MD: Aspen Publishers, Inc.

Zaleznik, A. (1981). Managers and leaders: Are they different? *Journal of Nursing Administration, 11,* 25–31.

Ziglar, Z. (1986). *Top performance.* Old Tappan, NJ: Berkley Publishing Corporation.

Recommended Readings

Garfield, C. (1986). *Peak performers: The new heroes of American business.* New York: Avon Books.

King, P. (1987). *Never work for a jerk.* New York: Bantam Doubleday Dell Publishing Group, Inc.

Roane, S. (1989). *How to work a room.* New York: Warner Books, Inc.

Robbins, A. (1986). *Unlimited power.* New York: Ballantine Books.

2

ORGANIZING AN AUDIOLOGY AND SPEECH-LANGUAGE PATHOLOGY (ASLP) DEPARTMENT IN A HEALTH CARE SETTING

David W. Stein, PhD and
Karen G. Stein, MA

"*All glory comes from daring to begin.*"
(Eugene F. Ware, American Lawyer/Poet)

An effective Audiology and Speech-Language Pathology (ASLP) program must have a well defined mission. If the program is part of a larger health care organization, that mission must be consistent with the mission of the larger organization that it serves. The program must be capable of meeting the needs of its many customers, whether those are patients, administrators, or other professionals. As the needs of the customers change, there must be a corresponding change in the way the department is organized and in the way services are provided. In today's work environment, department managers have limited resources to meet their goals. They must continually search for the most effective approach to generate revenue, using an organized process that distinguishes the role of the ASLP department in the organization. This chapter will examine the activities that all managers must be cognizant of in carrying out their responsibilities, regardless of the size of the staff, the nature of the organization, or the range of professional services offered.

ESTABLISHING AN ASLP DEPARTMENT

There are several ways to establish an ASLP department where none currently exists. Top management usually makes the decision that a department is to be established, but situations still exist in which you will have the opportunity to approach them and sell them on the idea. To determine the responsibilities to be assigned to the new department manager, the top executives may hire an outside consultant to provide guidance concerning the scope of services to be offered, or they may send a representative to visit similar organizations. The newly hired manager may be fortunate to select from a cadre of clinicians to formulate the core of the new department. The basic components of an ASLP department are: (1) the staff clinicians who actually treat the patients; (2) the managerial staff; and (3) the supporting clerical staff. As the size and complexity of the department increases, the department manager will have to hire or promote supervisors to coordinate activities within the clinic. The addition of supervisors represents the first division of labor beneath the department manager. This division makes a distinction between those who treat the patients and those who supervise the staff. The department manager, who is in middle management with respect to the total organization, is ultimately responsible for supervising the entire staff. The program administrator is positioned between the staff and top management. It is top management that guides the destiny of the organization, its strategic planning, and determines the activities necessary to achieve its objectives. Regardless of the size of the ASLP department or the type of enterprise involved, all departments have a number of functions in common. These functions determine how the department will accomplish its mission (Dressler, 1976). A simplified diagram showing the responsibilities and work flow generated by traditional ASLP departments is shown in Figure 2–1.

The past 30 years have seen significant changes in the responsibilities normally assigned to ASLPs. These changes are the result of an ever-increasing body of knowledge concerning the clinical aspects of hearing, speech-language, and balance disorders, and technical advancements that have brought ASLPs into neurodiagnostic and advanced rehabilitation

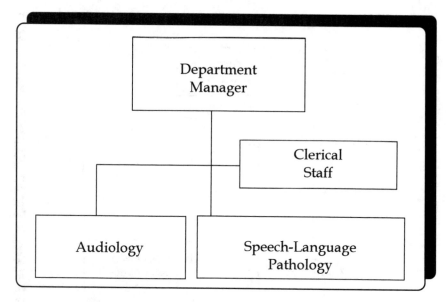

Figure 2–1. Simplified functional diagram of an audiology and speech-language pathology department.

environments. This knowledge base has been a prime reason for restructuring the services provided by the traditional ASLP program (Figure 2–2).

There is another organizational design that is available to ASLP departments that employ a large staff. This alternative utilizes specialty groups (grouped by function) within the department. A technical specialty is assigned to employees who, by virtue of academic training, experience, personal interest, or clinical research, have elected to become experts in a specific area. These specialists are then assigned to clinical teams on the basis of the specific skills required to evaluate and treat a given type of patient. The use of organization by function is likely to increase in the future (Coile, 1990), as departments must justify their operational costs for clinical services. It is a straightforward way to determine how much it costs to deliver a clinical service. The intent here is to maintain profitability in a era of declining revenues.

ORGANIZATIONAL DESIGN

Organizational charts are graphic representations that display the relationships between an organization and its members. As an ASLP department grows, the need to divide and coordinate the activities of its members increases. If the ASLP department is small, the administrator will typically perform clinical work as well. In larger departments, the program administrator will advise or oversee the entire staff of supervisors who will oversee the clinicians (Figure 2–3). This is referred to as *line/staff* organization. Here,

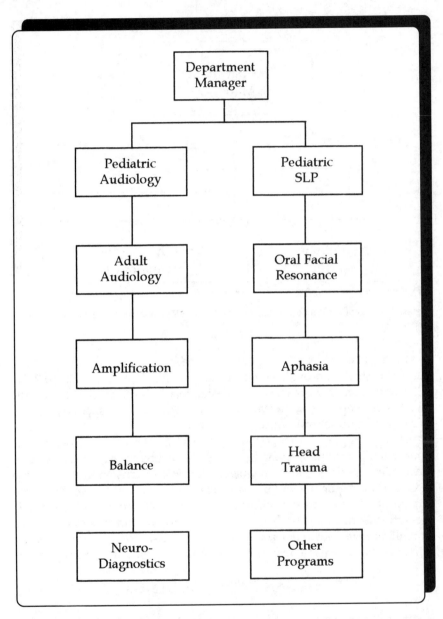

Figure 2–2. Functional diagram of an audiology and speech-language department restructured according to the services provided.

the department has expanded to a point where supervisors are needed to achieve increased efficiency of operation. Because of the presence of the supervisor (an additional layer of personnel), the response time for decision making increases. Line/staff organization designates activities, subdivisions,

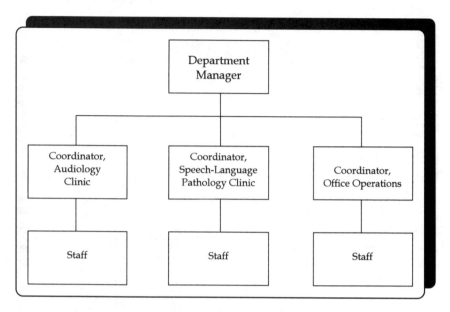

Figure 2–3. Line/staff organizational diagram of an audiology and speech-language pathology department.

levels of management or supervision, and lines of authority within an organization (Hellriegel & Slocum, 1986). Most health care organizations have an extensive line organization diagram that displays the intricate relationship between top management and its subdivisions (Figure 2–4). As seen in this illustration, clinical departments are separated from nonclinical departments that support the health care mission (Dressler, 1976).

Another design that may best suit the unique needs of a complex organization is the matrix design (Longest, 1990). Here, specialists are assigned to a particular work unit or interdisciplinary team away from their work site. For example, clinical activity underway in a particular location could require the assistance of various specialists (Figure 2–5). In this example, a clinician may report to the unit supervisor in stroke/neurology, head trauma, swallowing, or respiratory care. The unit supervisor is likely to contract for services in advance with a specific (by function) department manager. This allows the supervisor to obtain specialized clinical expertise while containing the cost for full-time staffing on that unit. This permits unit staffing to fluctuate with patient workload. In another example, ASLPs may be assigned to an interdisciplinary treatment team (such as a cleft palate team) that reports to a team leader. The formation of interdisciplinary teams can help to resolve the territorial disputes that may arise among professionals employed in different departments under traditional line organization structure (Michael et al., 1991).

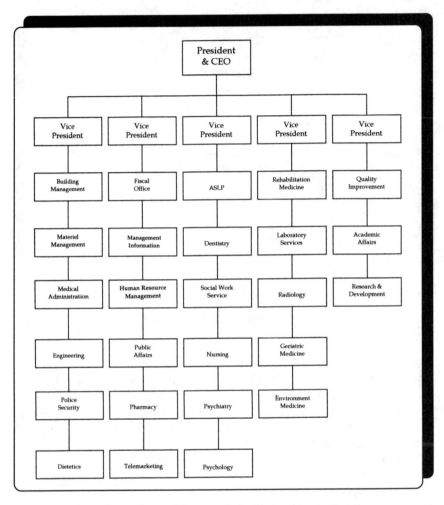

Figure 2–4. Line/staff organizational diagram of a health care organization.

Matrix organization appears to be most appropriate when professionals work in a changing, dynamic environment. Once the objective of these matrix units is accomplished, they may be eliminated. The matrix approach has several advantages: (1) it allows individuals to showcase their talents and to stay current in their area of expertise; (2) specialists may present their work at conferences or publish their findings in recognized journals; (3) each specialist tends to network with other professionals with similar clinical interests; and (4) these individuals serve as excellent resources to other staff and to graduate students, and they also make good continuing education instructors. Although these qualities may exist to some extent in any organizational design, a matrix design can be extremely productive when a group of specialists interact on a specific task.

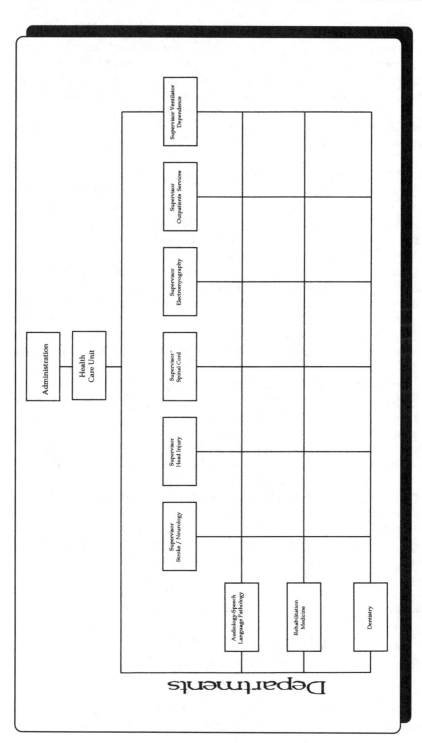

Figure 2–5. Matrix design of organizational function.

The disadvantage of matrix design is that the overall effectiveness of the primary supervisor and department manager is usually reduced because the employee's work site is away from the central department (Huse, 1980). A fundamental concern raised by specialists employed in matrix-type organizations is that they may have to answer to more than one superior concerning job performance issues (Michael et al., 1991). Because of the two-boss structure, the professionals within the matrix structure may face conflict because of the possibility of unclear expectations and priorities (Timm & Wanetik, 1983). Professional roles may need to be redefined and the concept of interdisciplinary functioning promoted (Darling & Ogg, 1984).

Another organizational alternative is exemplified by large ASLP firms which operate national headquarters and regional branch offices (Figure 2–6). The ASLP industry has recently utilized this approach because of trends in consolidation of clinical services. *Consolidation refers to the ability of a single provider to meet the primary, secondary, tertiary, rehabilitative, and custodial care needs of all patients in need of those services within a specific geographic region* (Nosse & Friberg, 1991). A primary question is how much decision making should be done by corporate management and how much should be left to each division. Organization by location has the advantage of increased economy and efficiency. The primary disadvantages are decreased central control and potential duplication of services from region to region (Hellriegel & Slocum, 1986).

Duplication of services can be reduced through the development and coordination of services at the central headquarters. This requires the use of centralized policies and procedures for use by all branch offices. The more centralized the decision-making process becomes, the more time it takes for a decision to be made and the less responsive each division will be to external forces. From these examples it is evident that the organizational design can be uniquely tailored to meet the needs of any ASLP department. The direction that a new manager may take is dependent on the purpose and mission of the department with respect to that of the entire health care organization. Using the organizational design of another ASLP department may not prove to be the best approach in all cases; yet an awareness and understanding of organizational structure in other facilities may provide examples that might not otherwise be considered. The department's structure should be flexible to adapt to changes taking place in the environment of ASLP service delivery.

THE DEPARTMENT'S POSITION IN THE HEALTH CARE ORGANIZATION

During the initial interview, the prospective manager should ask about the position of the ASLP department within the parent organization. The purpose is to determine if the manager will have the authority to com-

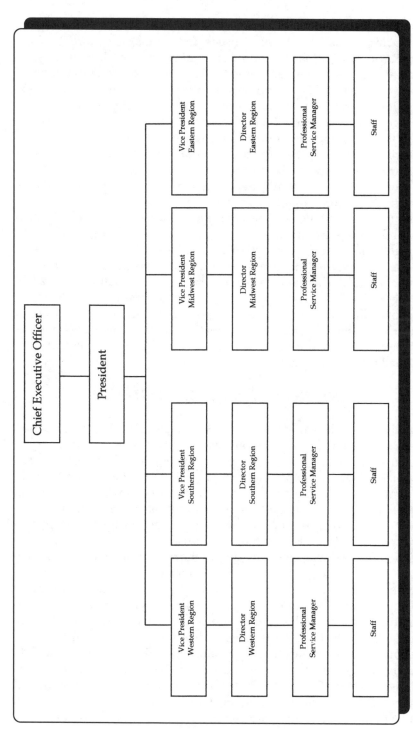

Figure 2–6. Location design of organization function.

municate directly with top management on issues related to the department's mission such as resource needs and standards of care. In some organizations, ASLP is a section within neurology, otolaryngology, or rehabilitation medicine departments. Any reduction in the number of layers between ASLP and top management will reduce the need for using intermediaries to speak on the behalf of the department. As the distance is increased between the department and top management, the ability to communicate with the primary decision makers diminishes. This follows, in part, the inverse square law which states, "as the distance from the source is doubled sound power decreases by 6 dB." The key word is power. Typically, department managers have little involvement in the positioning of their programs in the organization. In one example, the ASLP department is positioned between a university hospital and a university medical school (Figure 2–7). Although both establishments maintain administrative authority over the department, their expectations may not necessarily be the same. For example, university hospitals place greater emphasis on providing direct patient care, while the medical school places greater emphasis on research and teaching functions. Thus, it becomes difficult to serve two masters. Managers in this situation must balance institutional expectations, and possibly create release time opportunities for their staff to prevent burnout, stagnation, and turnover (Benner, 1984).

DEVELOPING A MISSION STATEMENT

Essential to the development of an ASLP department is a set of values that identify its purpose. This purpose is commonly referred to as the *mission statement*. Developing a mission statement means seeing a pattern that will get the department moving, assessing the resources available, and then formulating those ideas into words. The mission statement should be clearly described in terms that are easily understood and accepted by top management as well as by the other customers served. The mission statement describes the present and future direction of the department, and its commitment to excellence (Dailing, Pope, Stoltz, & Samuel, 1991). The professional contributions of the individuals within a department should be in alignment with the mission of the department. The more opportunities the manager gives the staff to align their mission with the department's own, the more likely the program is to succeed. The department's mission should complement the mission of the entire health care organization. This approach will align department values and standards of care with the objectives of the parent organization. For an ASLP department to be successful, it should continuously reevaluate its mission statement. In the absence of a mission statement, even an established program with a successful track

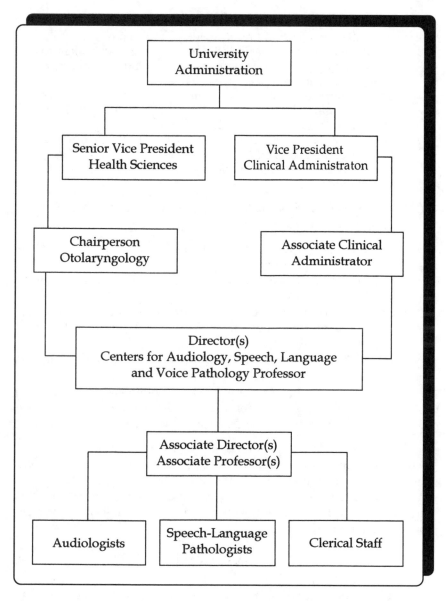

Figure 2–7. Dual university hospital and medical school design of organizational function.

record can experience decay within the organization. An example of a mission statement is as follows:

The Audiology-Speech-Language Pathology Department is a (1) for-profit organization, (2) dedicated to becoming a widely recognized provider of quality care, (3) provider of inpatient and outpatient ASLP services to, (4) persons residing in the Anywhere metropolitan area. In addition to the, (5) provision of ASLP services the department shall provide, (6) specialized treatment to adult and pediatric patients with peripheral and central disorders of the hearing and speech mechanism. The department is also (7) committed to meeting the continuing educational needs of the ASLP staff; the department will host professional meetings and maintain affiliations with accredited ASLP programs. All experimental and clinical research conducted within the ASLP department shall reflect a recognition of the basic dignity and rights of all employees, patients, students, referral sources, and the community.

The numbered parts of the mission statement identify the following characteristics of the department:

1. It is a profit organization, inclined to take risk and the challenges of competition.
2. There is importance placed on earning a positive reputation in delivering quality services.
3–6. The specific functions of the department, the areas in which service excellence will be demonstrated, and the geographic focus are defined.
7. A positive attitude toward education and research activities is stated.
8. The attitude of the staff toward those within and external to the department is clearly defined. Respect for human dignity is a value all members of the department shall demonstrate.

The specific wording of a mission statement helps the department focus on objectives it most desires to accomplish. Attention to the client puts the department above its competition. The challenge of fulfilling a mission can strengthen a wide array of personal and professional characteristics including leadership, collaboration, communication, problem solving, and dedication.

SETTING GOALS

The goals and objectives for an ASLP department should be discussed in detail with the entire staff. Setting goals for a department without staff participation is destined to be an unproductive process. Active staff participation tends to assure a high level of cooperation and commitment from the staff.

The objectives developed by top management describe the short- and long-range goals of the entire health care organization. To effectively respond to these objectives, ASLP administrators must develop a set of departmental goals consistent with the organizational goals. To accomplish these objectives, managers must have access to staff members who possess both specific technical skills and creativity. In a newly formed department, the administrator should meet regularly with members of top management to develop an understanding of the organizational objectives and the desired outcomes. These discussions should produce a set of requirements that the ASLP administrator may then use as a guide in organizing the functions of the department. The most effective channel of communication between line/staff begins with the department manager's contact with the supervisors, then the supervisor's contact with the clinicians, and finally the clinician's contact with the patient. Effective communication must consider everyone's perspective in order to have total participation and acceptance of departmental issues. Otherwise, a skewed perception of the department could be generated among line/staff members. By requiring mandatory attendance at regularly scheduled meetings, the manager will be able to guide the entire staff toward the achievement of the goals of the department. Some staff members complain that the time of the meeting conflicts with their clinic schedule. Absenteeism at meetings will reduce the effectiveness of the department. To prevent this from happening, meetings should be held at a standard time (e.g., the third Friday of each month at 9 a.m.). Clinic schedules can then be adjusted to accommodate the meeting time.

Some individuals aloofly believe that their clinic specialty is more important than another specialty. This behavior creates dissension among staff members, and may prove to be an insurmountable problem if not extinguished. Only through effective team building can a new department be created or existing one strengthened. This approach will create a firm foundation for assessing the department's present status and for improving its effectiveness to the clients served. If open communication is maintained, the image of the department will uniquely serve the parent organization. So place the emphasis on *we* and not *me*!

SELECTING MANAGERS AND SUPERVISORS

Managers should hold a graduate degree in ASLP with advanced training in program management. Equally important, managers should have training or experience in computer technology, the single most important cost-cutting instrument used in management. The qualifications of the ASLP administrator should meet the same high standards as those established for other department managers within the parent organization. The strength of the line/staff relationship is at stake. The staff should not be a refuge for second-class managers. In many cases, the in-house promotion of a staff member to department manager occurs to offset interviewing and relocation expenses. This approach has, unfortunately, created an era of professional consanguinity within many departments.

The position of the department may not improve if it only has its past staff to model after. Typically, clinical supervisors are selected from within the department. This would be the natural career path for the outstanding clinician who has an interest in administration. Every manager should establish a well-planned training program for developing new supervisors as early as possible. There are excellent programs developed by management consultants, outside agencies, and university training programs to prepare the staff for increased leadership responsibilities.

RECRUITMENT OF STAFF

Policies regarding the recruitment of professional staff are established by the Human Resource Management Department in most organizations. Some facilities utilize personnel officers to recruit all professional personnel, while others leave this responsibility to the department managers. Regardless of the practice followed, the mechanism for hiring ASLP personnel should occasionally be reviewed to ensure that the process fulfills the need to attract qualified personnel. For a more in-depth discussion on the topic of human resource management, the reader is referred to Chapter 4.

AFFILIATIONS

Affiliations with academic training programs can fulfill several needs and be beneficial to both institutions. ASLP departments housed in health care organizations have a very real need to stay abreast of current technology and changing clinical practices. Likewise, the first order of concern for university training programs includes the maintenance of relevant academic training and the provision for their students of clinical practicum opportunities. Managers may use their university affiliations as a conduit for personnel recruitment, to fulfill temporary manpower requirements via clinical practicum opportunities for graduate students, and also to satisfy their department's continuing education needs. Graduate schools are constantly looking for practicum sites that will enable their students to obtain clinical experience with a diversified caseload. These cooperative arrangements have proved to be most beneficial, and they have figured prominently in the training of most ASLPs.

DEVELOPING NEW TECHNIQUES AND SERVICES

ASLP administrators are obligated to stay current on issues that will have an impact on the department and the profession. This obligation is the key to professional survival. Any manager who fails to accept this responsibility is on the road to extinction. A failing department will create low employee morale, absenteeism, high turnover, and general frustration. Staff atrophy is an ailment that is costly to the department, and will eventually lead to its erosion. Staff members have the right to expect peak performance from their department manager and vice versa.

The past 30 years have seen an enormous increase in both the quantity and quality of information and educational programs available to the ASLP. Conferences on every conceivable concept or technique are conducted frequently, and within relatively easy reach of most facilities in North America. Publications in applied clinical research have also become more numerous and highly specialized during this time frame. The journals and proceedings of national and international conferences reflect the high standards required by the contemporary clinician. At the same time, there is a dearth of publications in allied health management and in leadership development for individuals with a career interest in administration. Managerial effectiveness and leadership ability can be enhanced by attending seminars conducted by professionals in health services management or offered by colleges with programs in health services/hospital administration.

GIVE PRIORITY TO WORK ASSIGNMENTS

The national effort to curb health care expenditures should change an administrator's perceptions of service delivery. The entire department must devote its efforts to increase productivity, meet future expectations, evaluate new technology, maximize reimbursement, and educate their various customers (top management, the medical community, and the consumer) about these changes. The manager must balance the unique objectives of ASLP when designing the department. Clinical services must be adequately priced to offset the operating costs of the department. This approach will result in a redefinition of certain services offered and will lead to the future development of alternative services. For some services, the prioritization is predetermined. Top management may issue guidelines up front, eliminating the need for departmental input. Other services may be eliminated by the department because of high cost, poor marketing, lack of technology, or poor return on an investment. In many instances, department committees are formed to determine which services should be staffed and to establish a priority list of services. The prioritized list of services includes estimates of their cost to the department and benefit to the consumer. Because of limitations in resources or limited technical skills available, some services will have to be eliminated to accommodate those services with greater potential or with a higher degree of importance.

SUPERVISORY AND MANAGERIAL ROLES

ASLPs are usually grouped according to function under the direction of a clinic coordinator/supervisor. This individual assigns the work, advises the staff on equipment and procedures, reviews case studies, and reviews their annual performance. In today's workplace, the supervisor may serve as a resource to the department manager. The more traditional, sub-servient role is being reshaped by the increasing complexity of clinic func-tions, quality improvement issues, and the need to deal with more challenging administrative matters. More time is spent in paperwork management and less time in overseeing direct patient care activities. This satisfies the needs of the department manager by providing more assis-tance in strategic planning and decision making, and delegates more patient care responsibilities to the clinician.

Managers should be viewed as a resource to the department and to all levels of management within the parent organization. They must cre-ate and support vertical line/staff interactions within the department, as well as those that occur horizontally between specialties. Managers should be physically present, should manage by walking around, but should not serve as a referee to resolve personnel disputes (unless the department is without supervisory personnel). Department managers usually serve on committees that influence the future direction of the entire health care organization.

OTHER CONSIDERATIONS

Policies and Procedures

In establishing an ASLP department, the development of clear policies and procedures can serve a vital function by defining expectations and standards of performance. Policies and procedures are an organization's written rules and regulations that describe the values of the organiza-tion, defining specific directions, goals, and expectations (Kaluzny et al., 1982). A policy and procedures (P&P) manual can be used as a manage-ment tool and as a training aid for employees to avoid misunderstand-ing and errors. Rao (1991, p. 1) stated that a P&P manual is "required by accrediting, certifying, licensing, and regulatory bodies, such as the Joint Commission on Accreditation of Healthcare Organizations (JCAHO), the Commission on Accreditation of Rehabilitation Facilities (CARF), state licensing boards, state and local education agencies, and the Professional Standards Board (PSB) of the American Speech-Language-Hearing Association . . . a living document of policies and procedures that form the foundation of any service delivery program, whether it be in a school, private practice, hospital, or other health care setting."

There are many and varied procedures that can be followed in developing a P&P manual. The manual can be a compilation of submis-sions from many individuals. Policies and procedures can be combined or there can be a separate section for policies and a separate section for procedures. When these decisions are made, it is necessary to decide on the contents of the manual and develop a list of subjects to be covered. This list can then be divided into major topic categories.

Appendices 2A–E provide sample pages of tables of contents of P&P manuals for the reader's review. Of interest is the way the responsibilities for implementing certain parts of the procedure are defined, the coding system, and the dating of the procedures. It is important to remember that a P&P manual must continually be revised and maintained. Using a simple writing style and tailoring the manual to meet the department's needs will make the manual more effective. Although narrative style is common, the use of playscript format has proved more effective for some (Liebler, Levine, & Dervitz, 1984). Procedures should be written to reflect the most efficient method of carrying out a task. They should reflect current regulations and standards of relevant accreditation programs. All procedures must also have administrative and supervisory approval. They should be signed and dated with revision dates noted. A good discussion on the topic of P&P manuals was recently published by ASHA (Rao, 1991).

The Changing Face of Reimbursement

Current forecasts predict a further rise in the number of people who will be living to the age of 85 years and beyond. This has serious implications for all health care managers and providers, and will add to the existing difficulties they face in trying to provide a comprehensive system of health care. An ASLP department's competitive strategy is its plan for defending and taking a market share from its current and future competition. The relationship between a department's function, its product, and its marketability must be carefully evaluated to improve its posture in the marketplace. Restrictions imposed by governmental regulations on ASLP practice are found at federal and state levels. Governmental reimbursement for services is often contingent on the training and licensure of the provider. State licensure laws for ASLPs may place restrictions on organizational design. Licensure establishes standards for training and skill requirements and imposes restrictions on the service provider concerning patient care issues. Regulation of ASLP practices also comes from JCAHO and CARF, as described above.

The rising cost of health care has steadily changed the reimbursement structure of the entire service delivery system. Managed care plans are now becoming more common than traditional health insurance plans. The most common of these prepaid group hospital plans is the *health maintenance organization* (HMO). *An HMO is defined as "an organized system which provides an agreed upon set of comprehensive inpatient and outpatient health services to a voluntary enrolled population in exchange for a predetermined, fixed, and periodic prepayment"* (Berman, Weeks, & Kukla,

1990, p. 144). Most of the early HMOs began as non-profit group medical practices which required preapproval of services. Recently, HMOs have started to contract with existing hospitals for beds and services rather than build or buy them. Another option in prepaid health coverage is the *preferred provider organization* (PPO). *PPO contracts require the provider to submit a preset fee for services, with the incentive being that they will receive increased patient referrals* (Boland, 1985). Here, the provider gives the patient an acceptable reimbursement rate as full payment for services. If the provider submits a fee that is too high, then the PPO will not recognize them as one of their preferred providers. Yet another option is *self-insurance by the employer.* In this case, *the employer absorbs the cost of employees' health care, but has an insurance company or third party administrator process the claims.* These developments have forced traditional health insurance carriers such as Blue Cross/Blue Shield to also offer such options to remain competitive (Berman et al., 1990).

The reader is being provided this information because managed care plans may restrict coverage for ASLP services, or they may already have a contract with a specific provider (your competition). *If your organization does not participate in a particular plan, the patient is classified as uninsured and will have to absorb the cost for ASLP services.* The popularity of managed health care plans is changing the nature of health care reimbursement in this country. One such change is a national fee schedule for physicians, referred to as *resource based relative value scale. The fee is determined by the amount of work performed during a medical visit, the actual costs to the medical practice, and the costs of training the specialist who performs that service* (ASHA, 1992). This scale is being phased in by the federal government and other third party payers, and will likely replace the traditional payment system that is based on actual, customary, and prevailing charges (Coile, 1990). Initially, only ASLP services furnished as part of a physician's practice will be covered under this system. The ultimate impact on nonphysician services is thought provoking. A positive relationship between the ASLP department and the medical community will aid in its growth, financial independence, and future expansion.

National Health Insurance

The concept behind a national health insurance plan is to curtail rising costs and to provide care to many U.S. citizens who are without adequate health care coverage. In the past, national health insurance did not appear to be a strong issue. The Medicare experience convinced many that health care costs could not be controlled. However, the graying of America and the continuing spiral of increased health care costs have forced a national debate on the establishment of a national health insurance plan. Although the federal government has been unable to attain closure on this issue, the Clinton Administration is presently working to make this health care need a reality. Several states (e.g., Florida, Hawaii, Oregon, Vermont, and Washington) have developed their own health insurance plan. In 1992, Minnesota became the first state to offer comprehensive health care insurance to its residents. For example, a three member household with an aggregate income of less than ten thousand dollars would pay approximately ten dollars per month for comprehensive health insurance.

CONCLUSION

The ASLP department must have the mission of providing excellent care, and must carefully develop quality improvement measures to accomplish this objective. By building on your clinical and administrative strengths, and by developing a clear plan for the future, you can develop a model ASLP department. There are many factors for the ASLP administrator to consider when organizing a department. The topics discussed in this chapter will be influenced by being part of a larger organization and by external regulations imposed on ASLP practice. Organizational design may reduce the manager's ability to introduce the spectrum of services offered elsewhere. The manager must identify the restrictions imposed by the health care environment as well as the opportunities available to improve departmental operations. The correct organizational design is the first step toward this achievement.

REFERENCES

American Speech and Hearing Association. (1992). Strategies for responding to the medicare resource-based relative value scale (RBRVS). *Asha, 34,* 63–68.

Benner, P. (1984). *From novice to expert: Excellence and power in clinical nursing practice.* Reading, MA: Addison-Wesley.

Berman, H. J., Weeks, L. E., & Kukla, S. F. (1990). *The financial management of hospitals.* Ann Arbor, MI: Health Administration Press.

Boland, P. (1985). *The new health care market: A guide to PPOs for purchasers, payors, and providers.* Rockville, MD: Aspen Publishers, Inc.

Coile, R. C. (1990). *The new medicine: Reshaping medical practice and health care management.* Rockville, MD: Aspen Publishers, Inc.

Dailing, D., Pope, M., Stoltz, P. K., & Samuel, M. (1991). Team performance: The critical factor in continuous quality improvement efforts. Chicago, IL: American Hospital Association.

Darling, L. A., & Ogg, H. L. (1984). Basic requirements for initiating an interdisciplinary process. *Physical Therapy, 64,* 1684–1686.

Dressler, G. (1976). *Organization and management: A contingency approach.* Englewood Cliffs, NJ: Prentice-Hall.

Hellriegel, D., & Slocum, J. W. (1986). *Management* (4th ed.). Reading, MA: Addison-Wesley.

Huse, E. F. (1980). *Organization development and change* (2nd ed.). St. Paul, MN: West Publishing Co.

Kaluzny, A. D., Warner, D. M., Warren, D. G., & Zelman, W. N. (1982). *Management of health services.* Englewood Cliffs, NJ: Prentice-Hall.

Liebler, J. G., Levine, R. E., & Dervitz, H. L. (1984). *Management principles for health professionals.* Rockville, MD: Aspen Publishers, Inc.

Longest, B.B. (1990). *Management practices for the health professional.* Norwalk, CT: Appleton & Large.

Michael, L. E., Hagerman, E. J., Kerman-Lerner, P., LeDuc, J. A., Pietranton, A. A., Frattali, C. M., & Carey, A. L. (1991). An introduction to product line management. *Asha, 33,* 61–63.

Nosse, L. J., & Friberg, D. G. (1991). *Management principles for physical therapists.* Baltimore, MD: Williams & Wilkins.

Rao, P. (1991). The policy and procedure manual: managing "by the book." *Quality Improvement Digest,* Fall. Rockville, MD: ASHA.

Timm, M. M., & Wanetik, M. G. (1983). Matrix organization: design and development for a hospital organization. *Hospital Health Services Administration, 28,* 46–58.

APPENDIX 2A

P & P Manual Table of Contents—Sample

Besides revealing what is in a P&P manual, a table of contents shows how the material is organized. The following table of contents is from the policies and procedures manual of the Audiology and Speech Pathology Service, Department of Veterans Affairs, Chillicothe, Ohio, submitted by Stephen R. Rizzo, Jr., PhD. The service offers the full complement of routine and specialized diagnostic procedures to in-patient and outpatient veterans who are eligible for treatment. This example shows a clear and logical organization of a P&P manual.

The reader should note the decimal coding system that identifies the procedures. The use of such a system is a layout that is most flexible. A narrative writing style is used when preparing written policies.

APPENDIX 2B

Safety Practices Memorandum—Sample

The following safety practices service memorandum is adapted from the Audiology and Speech Pathology Service, Department of Veterans Affairs, Chillicothe, Ohio.

AUDIOLOGY-SPEECH   DVA MEDICAL CENTER
PATHOLOGY SERVICE   CHILLICOTHE, OHIO
MEMORANDUM NO. 126-05   June 17, 1993

AUDIOLOGY & SPEECH PATHOLOGY SERVICE SAFETY PRACTICES

1. PURPOSE: To establish Audiology-Speech Pathology Service Safety practices.
2. POLICY: To promote awareness of safe practices to meet the needs of all eligible veteran patients and to assure that the services provided are consistent with acceptable levels of standard and safe clinical practice.
3. RESPONSIBILITY:
    a. The service chief is responsible for safe work practices and will address and correct any unsafe conditions or practices through training, investigation, provision of protective clothing and supplies. Employees are responsible for preparing written accident reports within 48 hr of the incident.
    b. Employees are responsible for providing safe work practices and will receive a minimum of 4 (four) hr of mandatory in-service safety training.
4. PROCEDURES:
    a. Office Safety:
        (1) Employees must keep all floors, aisles, and exits free of spills, ice, debris, and so forth.
        (2) Employees are responsible for knowing the location of fire exits, fire extinguishers, and fire alarm boxes.
        (3) Employees must close all drawers of desks, filing cabinets, and so forth, immediately after use.
        (4) Sitting on the edge of chairs equipped with casters or balancing on two legs of a chair is prohibited.
        (5) Office machines will be placed so that electric cords do not obstruct aisles or passageways.
        (6) Contents of file cabinets will be arranged so that the load is distributed equally throughout the entire cabinet, rather than in the top drawers.
        (7) Materials will not be piled on the top of file cabinets nor stacked on the floor.

(8) Employees will report all office furniture in need of repair to the service chief.

b. Biomedical and Electrical Equipment Safety:

(1) Employees are responsible for notifying Engineering Service of all damaged electrical cords, plugs, and switches.

(2) Employees will terminate all equipment and instrumentation prior to the close of business day and prior to cleaning.

(3) Engineering Service will inspect personally owned appliances prior to usage and periodically thereafter.

c. Chemical Safety:

(1) Audiologists must use eye protection when mixing earmold impression material or when modifying hearing aid earmolds.

(2) Employees are responsible for contacting the Fire Station when a toxic odor is detected and for initiating evacuation procedures.

(3) Material Safety Data Sheets (MSDS) are posted in the Secretary's work area.

d. Accident Prevention:

(1) Employees are cautioned to be observant of wet floor surfaces and are urged to notify Environmental Management Service if there is need for cleanup. Other objects such as wood, metal, stones, and torn rugs or mats, are safety hazards and must be reported even though they may appear to be minor in nature.

(2) Employees must use handrails when going up or down stairs and use caution when carrying materials in order to avoid slipping, tripping, or missing a step.

(3) Employees will assume the squat position when lifting objects close to the body and will never bend over to pick up anything. Employees will request assistance to lift heavy items.

(4) Employees will utilize escort services to assist in maneuvering patients in wheelchairs or on bed gurneys.

(5) Employees will utilize disposable plastic gloves during examination of the patient.

(6) Audiologists will use sharpened knives and drill bits only and will make cuts away from the body.

e. Fire Prevention and Fire Procedures:

(1) Employees will know the location of fire extinguishing equipment and accessible escape exits in the vicinity of the Audiology-Speech Pathology Service.

(2) Employees will evacuate their patients during all fire drills. Designated employee(s) will contact extension 444, turn off unnecessary electrical equipment, close doors and windows, and vacate via posted routes.

(3) Employees will evacuate their patients during fire emergencies. Designated employee(s) will activate the fire alarm system, contact extension 444, turn off all electrical equipment, close

doors and windows, extinguish small confined fires, direct fire personnel, and vacate following posted routes.

f. Recognize and Respond to Unsafe Conditions:

(1) Teamwork is essential in recognizing safety and documenting health hazards. Employees are encouraged to provide recommendations to the service chief at monthly staff meetings. The Occupational Safety Health and Fire Protection Regulations Handbook, located in the Secretary's work area, is available for employees' perusal.

(2) The Chief, Audiology-Speech Pathology Service will provide instruction to all new employees on the requirements of this memorandum.

g. Safety Education Plan:

(1) Subject matter experts will provide, upon request by the service chief, additional training at monthly staff meetings. Employee training records will be maintained and submitted to the Education and Training Office.

(2) The service copy of the Station Disaster Plan is located in the Secretary's work area. Employees will receive annual in-service training in this area to familiarize themselves with this document. The Disaster Drill consists of a 1 (one) minute blast, followed by a 30 (thirty) second silence period, followed by a 1 (one) minute steady blast.

(3) Employees will receive annual in-service training in the use of specific utility systems with steps to be followed in the event of their partial/complete breakdown. These procedures are outlined in Policy Memorandum No. 138-4, Utility Management Program. The utility systems include (but are not limited to):

(a) communication systems (i.e., telephone systems, computer systems, radio paging system, overhead paging system, fire alarms, exits, and extinguishers);

(b) electrical distribution/emergency power systems;

(c) elevators; and,

(d) plumbing systems.

(4) The service copy of the Station Medical Emergencies Plan is located in the Secretary's work area. Employees will receive annual in-service training in this area to familiarize themselves with this document.

(5) Employees will be assessed annually to determine their need for training on the use and maintenance of all equipment and instrumentation used in the Audiology-Speech Pathology Service that is applicable to their position description.

5. REPORTS: The monthly Safety Training Report is submitted to the Chairman, Safety & Fire Protection Committee.

6. REFERENCES:
     Joint Commission on Accreditation of Healthcare Organization Rehabilitation Services Standards, 1993.
     Occupational Health, Safety, and Fire Protection Regulations, DVA, Chillicothe, OH (unpublished manual).
     Audiology-Speech Pathology Service Infection Control Policy Service Memorandum 126-04.
     Audiology-Speech Pathology Service Policies and Procedures Manual, Safety Policies, Chapter 1, Section 1.24.
7. RESCISSION: Policy Memorandum 126-02, June 17, 1993. Chief, Audiology-Speech Pathology Service (126)

Distribution: Audiology-Speech Pathology Service Staff

APPENDIX 2C

P & P Manual, Table of Contents—Sample

John D. Durrant, PhD, Director, Center for Audiology and David W. Stein, PhD, Associate Director of the Center for Speech, Language, and Voice Pathology, University of Pittsburgh Medical Center, Pittsburgh, PA, have contributed the indices from their departments' policies and procedures manuals, along with sample pages. The University of Pittsburgh Medical Center has more than 1500 acute care, psychiatric, and physical rehabilitation beds. The Center for Audiology employs four full-time audiologists, three support staff, and two part-time audiologists. The Center for Speech, Language, and Voice Pathology employs four full-time speech-language pathologists (SLPs), one support staff, and two part-time SLPs.

Again, the reader should note that the index has a system for indicating when the procedures were written, updated, and reviewed. The reader should also be aware that policy number identifies the procedure that relates to the index and the system for reporting the procedure's history. The sample policies were written in abbreviated narrative and playscript styles, respectively.

EYE AND EAR INSTITUTE
Center for Speech, Language, and Voice Pathology
Finalized: October 1, 1990
Updated: October 1, 1991
Audit Date: October 1, 1992

INDEX

Policy number

ADMINISTRATIVE POLICIES
Policy #1:   Policy and Procedure Manual.
Policy #2:   Review of Policy and Procedure Manual.
Policy #3:   Review and Evaluation of Speech Pathology Services.
Policy #4:   Hours of Operation.
Policy #5:   Payroll Time Sheet Preparation (deleted, refer to hospital manual).
Policy #6:   Orientation of New Employees.
Policy #7:   Disaster Policy.
Policy #8:   Patient Incident Reports.
Policy #9:   Employee Incident Reports.
Policy #10: Telephone Procedure for Incoming Calls.

Policy #11:   Continuing Education.
Policy #12:   Employee Job Descriptions.
Policy #13:   Reporting Off From Work.
Policy #14:   Paid Time Off.
Policy #15:   Uniform and Dress Policy.
Policy #16:   Quality Improvement Plan.
Policy #17:   Staffing.
Policy #18:   Supervision of Noncertified Personnel.

CLINICAL PROCEDURES—SPEECH-LANGUAGE PATHOLOGY

Policy   #1:   Evaluation of speech, language, and voice disorders.
Policy   #2:   Treatment of speech, language, and voice disorders.
Policy   #3:   Speech and voice tape recordings.
Policy   #4:   Evaluation and management of tracheostomy patients.
Policy   #5:   Management of nonvocal patients.
Policy   #6:   Inpatient loan of an electrolarynx.
Policy   #7:   Short-term loan of an electrolarynx.
Policy   #8:   Long-term loan of an electrolarynx.
Policy   #9:   Repair of electrolarynges.
Policy #10:   Sale of an electrolarynx.
Policy #11:   Bedside evaluation and treatment of patients with swallowing disorders.
Policy #12:   Evaluation of dysphagic patients using a modified barium swallow.
Policy #13:   Fitting of voice prostheses.
Policy #14:   Videoendoscopic/Videostroboscopic procedures.
Policy #15:   Referral for audiological service.
Policy #l6:   Cognitive assessment and retraining.
Policy #17:   Specialized equipment.
Policy #18:   Deep suctioning ventilator patients.

CLINICAL MANAGEMENT POLICIES

Policy   #1:   Indications for referral.
Policy   #2:   Admission procedures.
Policy   #3:   Relationship of speech pathology to other hospital services.
Policy   #4:   Ordering of supplies.
Policy   #5:   Petty cash.
Policy   #6:   Infection control.
Policy   #7:   Infection control for patient devices.
Policy   #8:   Patient infection control.
Policy   #9:   Patient supplies.
Policy #10:   Medical direction.
Policy #11:   Release of Information.
Policy #12:   Patient consent.

Policy #13:   Record retention.
Policy #14:   Notification of patient cancellations.
Policy #15:   Medicare patient re-certification for therapy.

SAFETY POLICIES

Policy #1:   Fire Procedures
Policy #2:   Explosive and electrical hazards
Policy #3:   Emergency drug box and emergency equipment
Policy #4:   Examination of seriously ill patients
Policy #5:   Patient safety

CLINICAL PROCEDURES—CENTER FOR AUDIOLOGY

Policy #1   Pure Tone Audiogram Air Conduction
Policy #2   Pure Tone Audiogram Bone Conduction
Policy #3   Speech Audiogram (Speech Reception Threshold and
               Speech Understanding Testing)
Policy #4   Pure Tone Stenger Screening Test
Policy #5   Pure Tone Stenger Test for Identification of Threshold
Policy #6   Modified Speech Stenger Test
Policy #7   Doerfler-Stewart Test
Policy #8   P-B Rollover
Policy #9   Olsen-Noffsinger Tone Decay Test
Policy #10   Masking Level Difference Test
Policy #11   Modified High Level Short Increment Sensitivity Index (SISI)
Policy #12   Procedures for Testing Children
Policy #13   Visual Response Audiometry
Policy #14   Conditional Play Audiometry
Policy #15   Impedance Audiometry
Policy #16   Cochlear Implant Testing
Policy #17   Evoked Potential Testing
Policy #18   Hearing Aid Evaluations
Policy #19   Delivery of a Hearing Aid
Policy #20   Taking Earmold Impressions
Policy #21   Repairing Hearing Aids
Policy #22   Return of a Hearing Aid
               American Speech-Language-Hearing Association
               Guidelines American National Standards Institute (ANSI)

APPENDIX 2D

Clinical Procedures—Sample

INDEX: CLINICAL PROCEDURES

SUBJECT: BEDSIDE EVALUATION AND TREATMENT OF PATIENTS WITH SWALLOWING DISORDERS

POLICY: The speech-language pathologist shall evaluate patients to determine the presence or absence of, and possible treatment for, oropharyngeal dysphagia.

PROCEDURES:

1. All evaluations are made on the basis of referral from a physician.
2. The medical history is reviewed, noting any dietary restrictions.
3. Nursing is notified of the potential need for suctioning during the examination (for inpatients).
4. A clinical examination is completed to determine the patient's cognitive status for swallowing, as well as therapy techniques, dietary management, and other compensatory strategies (such as positioning or the supraglottic swallow) that might benefit the patient.
5. If inefficient bolus transit or aspiration risk are indicated, the referring or case managing physician will be requested to order a modified barium swallow. This will be completed as a cooperative evaluation between the Radiology and Speech-Language Pathology Services.
6. The patient is visited subsequently for reinforcement of instructions, to reevaluate methodology and diet level, or to change strategies, as necessary.
7. Evaluation and follow-up therapy reports are recorded in the medical and/or speech chart.
8. Ongoing interaction with the physician, nursing staff, dietitian and family is essential.

Administrative Approval   Review Month

Date of Original Issuance   Department Chairman/Head

APPENDIX 2E

P & P for Ordering Supplies—Sample

CENTER FOR SPEECH, LANGUAGE, AND VOICE PATHOLOGY
DATE: October 25, 1992
SUBJECT: Ordering of supplies
POLICY: To assure that an adequate and updated supply of Speech
           Pathology materials and office items are maintained (within
           budgetary guidelines), supplies will be requisitioned through
           the storeroom or from distributors via Materiels Management.

RESPONSIBILITY	PROCEDURE
ASLP Staff	1. Periodically inventory supplies and order needed supplies via form (storeroom requisitions for purchase requisitions).
Director	1. Approve/disapprove of requisition and check budgetary guidelines. 2. Completes order forms as per samples using proper account numbers. 3. Keeps copies of all orders on file. 4. Forwards approved requisition to Materiels Management storeroom.
Storeroom	1. Fills/orders requested supplies and delivers to ASLP Department.
Director	1. Check delivered items with requisition, signs receipt, and updates inventory.

_____   _____

Administrative Approval   Review Month

_____   _____

Date of Original Issuance   Department Chairman/Head

3

PLANNING AND DESIGNING AUDIOLOGY AND SPEECH-LANGUAGE PATHOLOGY (ASLP) FACILITIES

Stephen R. Rizzo, Jr., PhD and
Jay E. Wilkins, PE

"We shape our buildings, thereafter they shape us."

(Winston Churchill, Prime Minister of England)

The delivery of ASLP services is undergoing considerable change. Administrators of large institution-based clinical programs who for decades were accustomed to treating captive markets have encountered an educated, value conscious, prosumer (client; customer) who prefers to receive services at convenient locations. The ASLP delivery system, in general, is being driven by several factors: (1) government stress on health care cost containment; (2) new technologies; (3) increasing competition in the health care marketplace; and, (4) a rapidly expanding aging population identified by physicians as needing ambulatory care (outpatient) services.

Faced with deficits and tight budgets, many hospital administrators have turned to well-managed, properly designed *ambulatory care buildings* (ACBs) to reduce both hospital-type construction costs and operating expenses compared to similar nonhospital facilities. By definition, *ambulatory patients are persons who can move about from place to place.* A prime reason one chooses an ambulatory care facility, over a hospital, is because the former is more easily accessible. ASLP clinics are ideally suited for ACBs, where additional health care services are needed, but where the duplication of large-scale hospital services are not a requirement. ASLP administrators, regardless of their place of employment, must realize the importance of thorough clinic planning and effective design to enable their staff to better achieve departmental goals.

The purpose of this chapter is to provide the reader with a process for planning and designing ASLP clinics. The end product of this process will serve as a tool that can be used by program administrators who work in a variety of health care settings. Before beginning the actual design process, a series of financial considerations must be discussed to relate them to the overall scope of the planning and design process.

TYPE OF OWNERSHIP

Several types of ownership (Halonen & Norville, 1987) have been described which can be used by hospitals in developing an ACB (that will eventually house the ASLP clinic).

Hospital-based Ownership

Perhaps the approach most commonly used is for the hospital to own and operate the ACB and receive the benefit from ultimate ownership. That is, the hospital provides ACB space and has complete control over the entire building. The hospital can identify the depth of ambulatory care services to be offered and can control the staff mix in each of the clinics. The primary disadvantage of this type of ownership is that the hospital has to obtain the capital for financing all of the health care programs. In many cases, ambulatory care services are provided in the hospital, but the ACB can also be adjacent to the hospital. In some cases, a hospital-based ACB can exist some distance away from the hospital.

Nonhospital Based (Affiliated)

An affiliated arrangement requires the hospital to finance and develop the ACB. The entire building is then sold to a third-party investor who leases the building back to the hospital. The hospital then subleases the building to professionals and assumes the responsibility for its management. However, for purposes of quality assurance and coordination, the ACB's staff, in part or whole, is provided through or by the hospital. This approach enables the hospital to maintain control over the building and staff through the monitoring of its quality improvement program. With this type of ownership, the hospital is devoid of the burden of financing the ACB (it gets its money back when the building is sold) but maintains control over its operation.

Nonhospital Based (Freestanding)

In a freestanding arrangement, the hospital finances the ACB and sells or leases it to a third party who then is responsible for its operation. The hospital also may lease space to a third-party investor who finances, develops, and manages all clinics under the requirements set up by the hospital in the lease. In a sale or lease arrangement, the hospital's interest is not protected to the same degree during the life of building as if it owned the clinics. With this type of ownership, the freestanding ACB has no financial or organizational responsibility to the hospital.

Other ACB entities can be sponsored by professionals who form a partnership or group corporation to own and operate the building. This approach can offer tax incentives to all professionals occupying space in the building.

ORGANIZATIONAL STRUCTURE

It is important to realize that there are several organizational considerations under which the ASLP may be established within an ACB. The arrangement chosen depends upon a number of factors in financing and in the type of ownership used (Halonen & Norville, 1987), such as:

- ∎ hospital-based institution;
- ∎ organized for non-profit;
- ∎ organized for-profit; and,
- ∎ a proprietary corporation.

Access to capital is a primary key to success in a competitive health care environment (Lightle, 1985). Most ventures for ambulatory care services do not require such a large investment in capital as compared to inpatient care services and therefore do not require substantial capital outlays. If the hospital were to establish an ACB according to the first type of arrangement, it would usually borrow money through a bond issue (Halonen & Norville). As a general rule, the bond issue prohibits the hospital from selling the ACB, any of its programs, or additional space to a for-profit corporation; therefore, the ACB becomes an extension of the hospital facility. One disadvantage of this approach occurs if patient revenues, which are the primary source of income, exceed expenses. Here, the portion of excess is used by the hospital to offset some of its expenses (otherwise known as Title V and Title XVIII expenses which represent the health care costs for benefits allowed by Medicare that are guaranteed under the Social Security Act) as part of the total hospital operation (Berman, Weeks, & Kukla, 1990). In other words, the federal government receives the benefit of the excess. If any of the programs operating in the ACB lose money, the hospital will have to subsidize those programs from patient revenue generated by other programs.

The second option is for the hospital to create the ACB program as a non-profit organization. However, if the revenue generated by ambulatory care services becomes substantial, it can adversely effect its tax-exempt status. The federal government will allow a non-profit organization to keep its tax exempt status as long as the non-patient revenues (e.g., rental space, barber shops, gift shops, parking, etc.) that it collects do not approach 50% of the total revenue (O'Brien, 1985). As a result, the hospital is allowed to have an excess of revenues over expenses, but it must use this excess as a partial offset against Title V and Title XVIII costs. The individual responsible for managing the ACB must keep abreast of changing legislation, regulated by the Internal Revenue Service, concerning unrelated business income.

The third option is to organize the ACB for profit. Thus, the ACB may be able to protect the excess of revenues over expenses that it earns. Moreover, the profit motive can give this excess to the hospital with no restrictions (imposed by the federal government) to be used for additional services the hospital wants to offer the public. This is after normal tax obligations for the for-profit organization have been paid. The for-profit status is a very desirable one as long the ACB is able to generate revenue in excess of its expenses.

Finally, a hospital may allow a for-profit corporation to house the ACB on hospital land. Unfortunately, this approach will cause the hospital to lose some of its control along with the advantage of obtaining the excess of revenues over expenses. However, if the ACB cannot generate the excess capital, but the hospital wants the convenience of having access to ambulatory care services, this may be the only alternative available.

These variations in financial concepts and the possibility of how ACBs may be sponsored by hospitals, physicians, and corporations should be carefully examined by prospective ASLP administrators seeking positions in these environments. This review should begin with an analysis of a number of factors including (but not limited to): financial control, availability of funds, ownership of land, and location. All of these factors must be considered in determining who will build and operate the ACB, and in determining the final organizational structure. This will have a significant impact on the major clinics and programs occupying the ACB.

ELEMENTS OF PROJECT COST

There are numerous activities that must be investigated when estimating projected costs for newly constructed facilities. While it may be uncommon for the ASLP administrator to have considerable involvement in the preliminary stages, this information is being presented to the reader to develop an insight into the process. Rostenberg (1986) and Halonen and Norville (1987) describe three major categories of project costs that must be considered:

■ **Direct Construction Costs**
  ● Building Costs. The cost of land (if not previously acquired), site development (e.g., excavation, backfill, and installation of utilities throughout the facility) construction, renovation (e.g., cost of structural changes, walls, floors, columns, and finishes, along with their labor costs), and landscaping. The occupancy date should be specified.
  ● Fixed equipment. Permanent equipment that is not a furnishing or a piece of moveable equipment (e.g., built-in audiometric sound suites are fixed equipment, while audiometers are considered moveable equipment).
  ● Utilities. Electrical, plumbing, heating, air conditioning, ventilation, and fire protection that are internal to the building may be critical in this period of rapidly escalating energy costs. The power requirements to be used in the building must be determined to arrive at a realistic estimate on a cost-per-square foot basis.
■ **Indirect Construction Costs**
  ● Management Costs. If an outside group owns the building, there may be additional costs of administration, housekeeping, landscaping, and building management. For example, these expenses would be incurred on a cost-per-square foot basis over a projected timeframe.
  ● Contractor's overhead.
  ● Furnishings. Furniture, draperies, carpeting, and so forth.
  ● Allowances. A predetermined amount which is usually a percentage of the direct construction cost is set aside for unforeseen conditions, such as increases in labor costs that may increase by the time the project is sent out for bid.
  ● Depreciation. An expense of doing business and is calculated by categorizing the total cost of the building and the equipment. These costs then are spread over the appropriate lifespan of the building and of the equipment and by rulings of the Internal Revenue Service as agreed to by both parties. For example, assume a construction cost of $3,000,000. Assuming

that the building is to be depreciated over 30 years and the ASLP equipment over 15 years, depreciation (the following calculations exemplify the straight line method of calculating depreciation; sum-of-the-years in digits and double declining depreciation are two other methods which can provide accelerated depreciation) would be structured as follows:

Total Construction Cost $3,000,000

Estimated 70% cost is building 2,100,000

Estimated 30% cost is equipment 900,000

Building life 30 years $\dfrac{\$2,100,00}{30 \text{ years}} = \$70,000/\text{year}$

*Equipment 15 years, $\dfrac{\$900,000}{15 \text{ years}} = \$60,000/\text{year}$

(*Depreciation for sound suites and similar systems; 5 to 7 years is more appropriate for electronic equipment. It is not because equipment wears out, but because it becomes obsolete.)

- Miscellaneous costs.

■ **Project Development Costs**

- Architectural and consultant fees. The architect's design fee is usually about 10% of the construction cost.
- Site survey.
- Insurance.
- Legal and accounting fees.
- Leasing and advertising.
- Financing. The method of financing the ACB depends on whether the program is owned by the hospital or by a proprietary group. If it is owned by the hospital, some hospital funds may be used to decrease the amount of borrowed money required to develop the ACB. However, if sufficient hospital funds are not available for the entire project, the balance must be financed during construction as well as over the life of the ACB.
- Permit fees. The cost for state-mandated regulatory reviews, building permits, and so forth.
- Taxes.
- Miscellaneous costs.

As more detailed information becomes available, tentative selection of space to house the ASLP clinic during the schematic design phase can be evaluated. After the ACB layout has been proposed and recommended for implementation by hospital management or the private entrepreneur, the owner of the building will select an architect or engineering firm to complete the planning and design phase. After the contract has been awarded to a particular company, a time schedule should be obtained that provides the completion dates of various construction stages. The architect/engineer will serve as the organization's representative in overseeing the contract during the construction phase. Any revision to the initial construction costs should be obtained in writing. The final estimate of all construction costs should be within 5% of the actual bid submitted by the contractor.

UTILIZATION OF SPACE

The decision to house the ASLP clinic in customized space is an important step in designing the ACB. Any specialized construction can affect the cost of the ACB which will have a significant effect upon the principal and interest payment of the debt ACB. If the owner decides to have sound suites imbedded in floor pits (ground level), financial arrangements with the other tenants must be established. For example, one option is to have ASLP clinic pay (e.g., private entrepreneur) for all extras. Another option is for the hospital to pay and build the cost into the ASLP lease agreement. To forecast expected revenues for ASLP, it is necessary to determine the rental value per square foot. (The authors note that elevated floors should be considered around sound suites which would permit similar access and can be easily removed for another tenant without major construction.) As previously mentioned, different rental rates could be established for specialty clinics based upon unique construction and design requirements (e.g., floor pits for audiometric sound suites or acoustically paneled rooms). If a hospital has a satellite ASLP clinic located in the ACB, additional revenue calculations are required. Rather than lease space to itself, the hospital usually handles such situations on a cost reimbursement basis. The first step in calculating anticipated revenue is to estimate the portion of space available for direct patient care for a designated period of time (e.g., three years). The space not used for direct patient care is assumed to be used for office operations and administrative purposes. To calculate the amount of rental space per clinician, it is assumed that the nonrent generating space is allocated on a proportional basis among clinicians. Therefore, each clinician is expected to generate enough patient revenue to cover a portion of the cost of this nonrentable space. For a discussion on the topic of financial management, the reader is referred to Chapter 8.

BREAK-EVEN ANALYSIS

Break-even analysis determines the point in operating a business when it produces neither a profit nor a loss (Snook & Ruck, 1987). This can be determined by analyzing the relationship between cost, volume, and profit. To achieve this objective, the ASLP administrator will have to separate costs into fixed versus variable versus semivariable components. Fixed costs remain unchanged despite changes in volume of activity. For example, if it costs $1000 per month to rent space for the clinic and 140 audiology evaluations are performed each month by one audiologist (e.g., 7 audiology evaluations per 8 hour day × five days = 35 evaluations per week × 4 weeks = 140 audiology evaluations per month), the cost for rent per evaluation is $7.14. If 150 evaluations are performed, the cost for rent per evaluation drops to $6.67. For the most part, from 20 to 40% of the costs of the new ASLP clinic may be *fixed (e.g., rent, air conditioning). These components are usually included in the basic part of the lease. Fixed costs have historically been attributed to depreciation, interest, and insurance.* These costs generally are fixed over the longevity of the ASLP clinic. *Variable costs refers to any cost that increases or decreases in direct proportion to the volume of activity.* In ASLP, the cost for *housekeeping and maintenance salaries are examples of variable costs.* The costs vary directly with the occupancy or use of the ACB. The more occupants in the ACB, the greater the cost. *Semivariable costs refer to those costs that are in part related to level of activity and the amount of time consumed. For example,* there is a cost associated with *having access to the telephone service.* There is also an additional cost associated with the use of the accessible telephone service. A portion of the cost would be incurred even if the telephone were never used. *Semivariable cost can be viewed as the cost of availability and usage* (Nosse & Friberg, 1991).

The ASLP administrator should note that once a desired occupancy level is determined for the entire ACB, the owners will attempt to stay at the break-even point by adjusting the rental schedule to match their cost line at the 90% occupancy level. That is, the lease agreement with the ASLP clinic, and all other occupants, will probably be designed so that the cost per square foot when the building is 90% occupied will allow the owners of the building to break even (Figure 3–1). For example, if the occupancy is less than 90%, the owners will suffer a loss. In most situations, the owners will usually include an inflation clause in the lease to cover inflationary costs that pattern trends in the economy (Halonen & Norville, 1987). Owners may also rent commercial space to clinics based on a percentage of gross sales. This arrangement will modify the break-even analysis. The break-even analysis is a very good management tool for the building owners, and occupants, to use to arrive at their break-even point and to estimate what will be needed in patient revenues (e.g., ASLP volume of activity) to cover their expenses. This can be used to determine the cash flow on a cumulative basis over time.

CERTIFICATE OF NEED

Many states require that the hospital (owner) of a proposed ACB submit an application to local governing agencies substantiating the need for such a facility. In theory, the purpose of the certificate of need is to

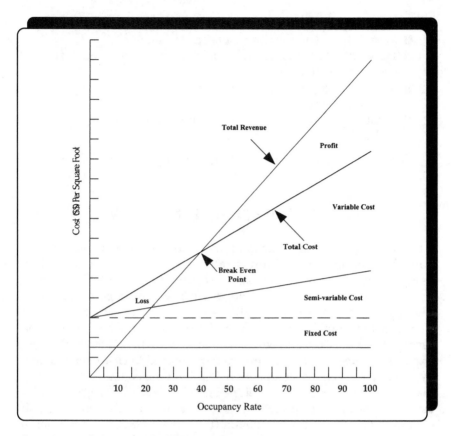

Figure 3–1. Ambulatory care building break-even analysis.

reduce unnecessary duplication of equipment and services, the cost of which would ultimately be passed on to the public. Because the regulatory agency has the authority to deny certification if it finds that a proposal is not in the best interest of the community, an experienced architectural consultant can be of great value during the review process (Rostenberg, 1986).

Clearly, developing the ACB is a complex business venture. Only through careful planning and prudent management during project development, and after completion, can the ACB become a valuable asset to a hospital or private entrepreneur in achieving its goals and serving its community.

CLINIC DESIGN

Once the decision has been made to establish the ASLP clinic, the administrator must ask the following questions:

- What impact will the clinic have on activity flow?
- What impact will the clinic have on staff morale?
- How will staff morale affect productivity, operating costs, and customer satisfaction?
- What impact will the layout design have on direct supervision within the clinic?
- What impact will the clinic have on its ability to adapt to change and satisfy future expectations?

These questions tend to highlight the importance of an effective clinic layout design.

SITE SELECTION

If the ASLP clinic elects to expand its scope of service in its present location, then the program administrator may proceed with the clinic design. However, when a new site is selected to deliver ASLP services, certain key issues must first be addressed. The most important issues in site selection are those relating to location and accessibility. The first step in determining a good location is to establish who the potential users of ASLP services are, where they live, and where they work. Other important issues in site selection are those related to customer availability, volume projections, competition, and building codes. A patient population model should be developed to simulate the projected ASLP market share for the future. Since there continues to be a significant shift toward the adult patient population (Fein, 1983, 1984), a redefinition of areas of patient concentration must be considered. It appears that these trends will continue well into the next century. As income levels continually change, one must take this into account not only for the present, but for future trends and projections. For an in-depth discussion on the topic of marketing, the reader is referred to Chapter 9.

Other important issues to consider are:

- Will the clinic be attractive and pleasant to draw future patients and staff?
- Will the clinic be located in areas where there may be language barriers associated with a potential ethnic and racial mix?

For the ASLP clinic to be a successful business venture, it is necessary to map the locations of competing ASLP clinics and of those health care facilities that might serve as future sources of patient referrals. In the race for patients and their communication health care dollars, it is desirable to map the entire ASLP network for the county, city, and state to see how the proposed clinic will fit into the existing delivery system. The age of ASLP competition is upon us. Community clinics, university clinics, urban and rural hospital-based clinics, and private entrepreneurs are vying for a portion of each dollar spent on communication health care each year in the United States. By keeping a vigilant eye on the competition, one can influence the proposed clinic's chances for financial success.

A well-designed ASLP clinic is of little value if it does not allow for easy access. People who travel great distances through either cumbersome rural routes or through large urban areas have different acceptable ranges of traffic congestion (Reizenstein, Grant, & Vaitkus, 1981). Ideally, the ASLP clinic should be located close to its patient population in distance and arrival time. Patients may be traveling only a few blocks from home, across town, from another city, or across the state. Therefore, calculations based on distance should be made in both miles and minutes. The ASLP clinic should be close enough to a major highway for easy access, yet not too close to be affected by noise pollution and traffic congestion (Lifton & Hardy 1982).

With such a large proportion of people arriving by car, adequate parking accommodations are important to attract prospective patients and qualified staff to the clinic. In calculating parking requirements, Allen and von Karolyi (1976) identify several questions to be considered:

- Who is expected to use the clinic (e.g., physicians, staff, patients and guests)?
- How many parking spaces will be needed for each group?
- What is the expected duration of the parking needs for each category of person?
- Will the clinic be open beyond the normal work shift?
- Will parking be on-site, along adjacent streets, or in existing parking lots? Will covered parking be provided? Will there be a charge for use of the parking area?
- Will staff and public parking be mixed or separated?
- Will there be separate parking spaces for audiology versus speech-language pathology patients?

Some of these issues can be answered by analyzing past and projected work load (e.g., the number, type, and duration of patient visits) to determine the number of parking spaces to be reserved for the ASLP clinic. Walking distances from parking lots should be kept as short as possible, and locations of lots should be integrated with respect to the location of the ASLP clinic within the ACB.

In some instances, health care organizations have attempted to recover the costs of providing a parking area. For the patient being seen for an initial audiological evaluation and a follow-up hearing aid evaluation, a standard parking fee appears reasonable. However, for the patient returning to the clinic for continuous treatment (e.g., speech-language-voice therapy) over a period of weeks or months, the standard parking fee may prove to be too costly. The ASLP administrator may not have much control over the parking fee schedule. In this case, long-term fees or free parking for patients and visitors, subsidized by adjustable rates charged to other users, might be a useful marketing game plan (Reizenstein, Grant, & Vaitkus, 1981).

For people utilizing public transportation, Carpman, Grant, and Simmons (1986) raise several questions that will need to be addressed, such as:

- Will patients have easy access to public transportation?
- Will the drop off area be close to the entrance of the ACB?
- Should the ACB be a satellite site of a primary hospital, and will people have access to a shuttle service?

Bus stops should be located close to the main entrance of the ACB. This will assist individuals in finding their way through the building and decreasing the distance they have to walk. When patients and visitors leave the building they need a safe, comfortable, weather-protected shelter in close proximity to the entrance of the ACB. A public transportation information system should be available to individuals using such a system (Reizenstein, Grant, & Vaitkus, 1981).

Once the ASLP site has been selected, a system for circulation through the ACB to the ASLP clinic must be developed for patients, staff, and visitors. The ASLP administrator should try to develop an effective and understandable sign system, as follows:

- Once the wording of the sign has been chosen, use it consistently (Carpman, Grant, & Simmons, 1986). Avoid using Audiology-Speech-Language Pathology Clinic on one sign and Speech and Hearing Department or Communicative Disorders Clinic on another.
- Signs should be visible to the driver directly and should be seen easily from behind the steering wheel (Folis & Hammer, 1979).
- Signs should be easily seen and within the viewer's 60-degree cone of vision (Folis & Hammer, 1979).
- Color combinations should be selected that are more visible than other colors. For example, black on white or black on yellow as opposed to red on white or yellow on red (Wechsler, 1979).
- Since 10% of the male population is color blind, avoid using color combinations of red and green (Wechsler, 1979).
- The letter size and typeface will have a direct effect on sign visibility. It is recommended (Carpman, Grant, & Simmons) that letters no smaller than 4 inches (10.1cm) high be used when speed limits are 30 to 35 mph and no smaller than 5 inches (12.7cm) where the speed limits are more than 40 mph (American Hospital Association, 1979).
- Outdoor signs should be visible during the day or night.

The placement of visual cues is an important consideration for alleviating congestion and confusion. The design of the circulation system should focus on visual cues created by the ACB and the surrounding landscape, because people often depend on visual cues to find their way through a building. The Americans with Disabilities Act of 1990 mandates easy access to entrances, elevators, water fountains, rest rooms and parking areas associated with health care organizations. For obvious reasons, the ASLP facility must be accessible by handicapped persons (e.g., people in wheelchairs, people with mobility impairments, disorders in vision, hearing, speech, and mental disabilities). For a more comprehensive treatment on the topic of design for accessibility, many useful reference books are available (Folis & Hammer, 1979; Passini, 1977).

TYPES OF SPACE

A familiarity with terminology applicable to the parts of a building is a prerequisite to understanding the clinic design process (Rostenberg, 1986), for example:

- ■ Activity space refers to spaces used directly for patient care (e.g., diagnostic and therapy rooms).
- ■ Support space includes those spaces that directly assist the function of an activity space (e.g., waiting rooms, telephone booths, vending machines, storage rooms, utility rooms, closets, and bathrooms).
- ■ Administration space includes space used to house staff members when they are not performing direct patient activity (e.g., offices, conferences rooms, and clerical areas).
- ■ Net square footage is composed of all the functional spaces required to serve a program.
- ■ Net unassigned footage consists of all other spaces such as circulation areas, toilets, hallways, closets, and storage.
- ■ Total floor space is the total net assigned and unassigned space.
- ■ Efficiency ratio (net assigned space/total floor space) represents the relative efficiency of the floor plan.

The need for activity, support, and administration space is usually determined by the volume of workload activity. The key space requirements for a given workload-related activity is referred to as a workstation (Hayward, 1985). A workstation is the basic activity space required to perform a given task (e.g., audiometric sound suite, therapy room, clerical space, etc.). When designing the layout of the ASLP clinic, the primary goal is to maximize the opportunity to remain financially solvent while minimizing the cost of service delivery. An ASLP clinic that is too small cannot adequately perform needed services, yet one that is too large costs more to operate than it generates in revenue. The amount of revenue the clinic is able to generate is influenced by the proportion of activity space to support space to administration space.

DETERMINE KEY SPACE REQUIREMENTS

Space requirements must consider the interaction between staff, patients, equipment, ingress (entrance), and egress (exit) to determine the total floor space required. Table 3–1 lists ASLP space recommendations adapted from several sources (Veterans Administration, 1980; Carpman, Grant, & Simmons, 1986; Rostenberg, 1986; Nosse & Friberg, 1991). It is often helpful to assemble a written room-by-room functional space list. The written list is useful for noting functional room requirements, such as diagnostic and therapy rooms, and for identifying minimum allowable net square footage per activity, support, or administrative workstation. Space requirements are usually expressed in terms of net square footage (Mariotti, 1982), thus enabling the ASLP administrator to check the accuracy of the space estimates. By dividing each element into activity, support, and administrative spaces, one can visualize service area efficiencies.

Graphic sketch diagrams should be drawn of each room to visualize each activity (Figure 3–2). On these is indicated the activity room, location of equipment, furnishings (e.g., desks, tables, file cabinets, sinks, electrical outlets, power outlet strips, doorway clearance, intercoms, telephones, etc.), and their relationships to other rooms. A scale of one quarter inch to equal 1 foot is traditionally used. For large rooms, a 1/8 inch scale is appropriate (Tompkins, 1982). The net square footage needed for a single area is then multiplied by the number of areas performing similar tasks. This process is repeated for each area in both the audiology and speech-language pathology sections. Combining the total net square footage for each section will determine the total floor space required for the entire clinic. An allowance for aisles and access should include additional footage to both the length and width dimensions of each activity area. A simple rule of thumb to relate total floor space of the facility is typically based on the number of visits per activity. For example, the total net square feet can be multiplied by an appropriate factor (low = .434 to high = .586) to arrive at the visits that can be served by each area. These factors were obtained from room measurements of 12 health maintenance organizations (HMOs), or group practice facilities (Rostenberg, 1986), based on the number of visits per year, day, and hour.

The envelope of the ASLP clinic should be located in interior space because of the need for a controlled sound environment (Veterans Administration, 1980). This means away from main pedestrian areas, hallways, elevators, heating, ventilating, air conditioning systems, or any other noise generating systems. The use of digital equipment requires the facility to be located away from transformers, X-ray equipment, and other magnetic field generating equipment. Interior space will allow security controls to be

Table 3–1. Size recommendations for planning ASLP spaces.

SPACE	SIZE*	VOLUME - FUNCTION COMMENT
Parking	12ft wide	1 car with door fully opened plus space between cars.
	16 ft wide	1 van with wheelchair lift.
Reception	50	Per person.
Waiting space	15	Per person. Expect escorts. Total allocation is 1.5 × maximum number of annual visits.
Staff Offices	80–140	Per person, depending on whether there are files to house.
Department Head	100–150	Per person, depending on whether there are files to house.
Dictation Cubicle	20	Per person, desk, and chair.
Conference - Group Therapy Room	225	Staff meetings for more than 5 or for group therapy.
Prefabricated Audiometric Suite	260	1 sound suite per audiologist. If located in the basement, suites should be recessed in the floor by 6 5/8 in. Space should be available for otoacoustic emissions measurements.
Hearing Aid Room	200	Includes workbench(s), chairs, shelving, refrigerator, probe microphone system, and cerumen management equipment.
Sound Treated Balance Lab	260	Electronstagmography and posturography equipment, desk, chair, computer, shelving above workbenches.
Sound Treated Neurodiagnostic Suite	250–300	Multimodality testing. May also include EEG and EMG. If located in the basement, they should be recessed in the floor by 6 5/8 in.
Sound Treated Aphasia Room	85–125	Sound treated environment for language retraining. Space for table, chair, wheelchair, tape recorders. staff office(s) can be used, if they are sound treated.
Speech Lab	300	Includes shelves above workbench(s), chairs, speech-voice science equipment, computers, desk, and chair.
Storage		Based on 10% of the treatment space available.

* Except for parking, all figures relate to net square footage.

Source: **Adapted from** *Management principles for physical therapists* **(1st ed., p. 173) by L.J. Nosse &D.G. Friberg (1991), Baltimore, MD: Williams & Wilkins.**

implemented to protect the well-being of both people and property against burglary, theft, or damaging sensitive information areas (e.g., computer information systems).

A simulation of clinic events will aid significantly in estimating activity flow. A simple, concise, circulation system usually indicates a well-orga-

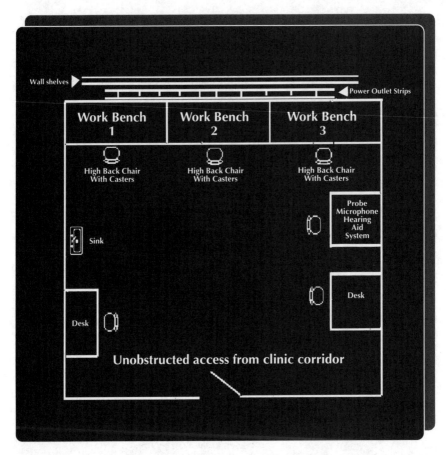

Figure 3–2. Graphic space diagram of a hearing aid room.

nized plan, whereas one with many confusing intersections indicates a less successful arrangement. The tentative location of each room within the clinic should then be reviewed, or modified as required, to obtain an integrated work area. Figure 3–3 shows how activity, support, and administrative space are designated relative to all other rooms in the clinic. An initial contact point (reception area and waiting area) is clearly visible from the point at which a patient first enters the clinic. A person entering the clinic is not confronted with many paths to choose from and is not likely to get lost. Internal staff flow is separated from patient flow. A separate staff entrance allows the ASLP staff to enter and exit the facility without passing through public zones. The appropriate arrangement of functionally related spaces can alleviate the problems of cumbersome activity flow and can be used by the ASLP administrator and architect to estimate projected cost and plan efficiency. Estimates of the total floor space required are usually based on criteria similar to those used to calculate a fee for service, namely:

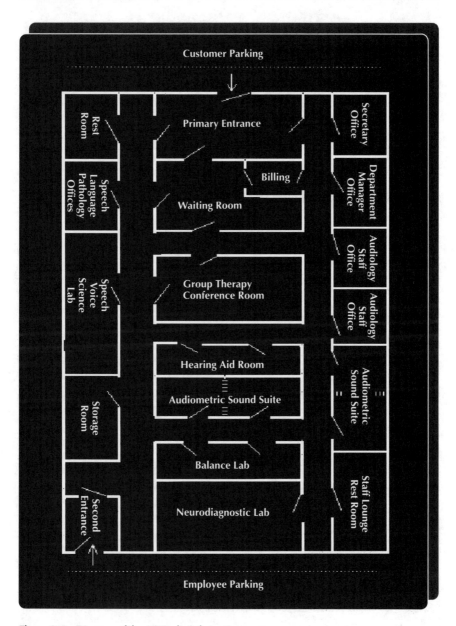

Figure 3–3. Diagram of the ASLP clinic layout.

■ Annual clinic visits per days open.
■ The distribution of routine and special ASLP clinical procedures that comprise the total number of visits.
■ Average length of appointment of each procedure.
■ Hours of operation.

■ The size and quantity of each unit of equipment.
■ Future growth expectations.

Rostenberg (1986) recommends collecting data specific to the above activity and recording the total values on a data collection form (Figure 3–4). This information forms the basis for determining the key space that is required for the ASLP clinic. For example, a previous annual work load of 5,040 routine audiology evaluations might imply a need for 3 to 4 sound suites in an ASLP clinic (e.g., 7 audiological evaluations per day × 5 days

Clinic: <u>ASLP</u>   Date:

Facility: <u>Anywhere Ambulatory Care Center</u>

Location: <u>Columbus, Ohio</u>

Owner: <u>Private Entrepreneurs of Ohio</u>

1. Type of Facility: _____ Freestanding _____ Attached to Hospital

_____

_____

_____

2. Projected Workload Indicators:

Type of Procedure   Number of Procedures per Year (Inc. Report)   Average Duration per Procedure

_____   _____   _____

_____   _____   _____

_____   _____   _____

_____   _____   _____

_____   _____   _____

Total Procedures per Year: _____

Average Duration per Procedures: _____

3. Projected Hours of Operation:

Operational hours per day _____   Procedures hours per day _____

Open _____   Close _____   Days open per week _____

_____Mon. _____Tue _____Wed _____Thu _____Fri _____Sat _____Sun

Operational days per year _____

Number of work shifts per day _____

Figure 3–4. Data collection form. (Adapted from: Bill Rostenberg Design Planning for Freestanding Ambulatory Care Facilities: A Primer for Health Care Providers and Architects.)

= 35 per week $\times$ 48 weeks per year $\times$ 3 sound suites = 5,040). These sound suites would create the need for an additional 500 net square feet of support and administrative space to accommodate additional audiologists.

SPATIAL RELATIONSHIPS

The level of interaction between ASLP and other specialties (e.g., Otolaryngology, Neurology, Optometry, Dental, Rehabilitation Medicine, etc.) signifies a necessary functional linkage between these functional areas based on urgency, convenience, and frequency of cross referrals. Therefore, a measurement of activity flow must be established. For example, one must determine if there is an absolute necessity that two clinics be close to each other, the importance of two clinics being close to each other, or the preference that two clinics not be close to each other. Interdepartmental spatial relationships within an ACB should consider the location of the aforementioned clinics in a wing of a building because of the likelihood of multiple sensory and motor disabilities among individuals and the opportunity for cross referrals.

DETERMINE ALTERNATIVE CLINIC SPACE

If the total clinic space required exceeds the net available space (total space minus corridors, elevators, and restrooms), then it is recommended that the total floor space must be reduced by considering the following options:

- Reduce the size of all rooms.
- Reduce aisle space and access space.
- Eliminate opportunities for further expansion.
- Eliminate space for future staff.
- Combine group therapy and conference room space.

The impact of these changes on staff productivity, marketability, and customer satisfaction must be considered. After the total floor space has been reestimated, the changes should then be summarized to reflect the alternative clinic plan. Since most ASLP clinics are located in renovated, existing areas, it is usually necessary to overcome existing problems while keeping the positive features of the existing area (Schmenner, 1979). The administrator may need to request additional space for expansion of ASLP services or staff or to increase productivity. These decisions will have a significant impact on the future expectations and long range goals of the clinic. The administrator must consider the following questions:

- Is the renovation temporary or permanent?
- How many patients are anticipated to be seen during this period?
- Which services are expected to expand or contract?

On the existing blueprint(s), the department manager and architect or project engineer should locate all permanent structures (i.e., columns, windows, doors, walls, ramps, fire alarms/exits, stairways, elevators, etc.). The size, length, and location of columns will determine whether the existing space is suitable to the needs of the department. Space selection should also consider the proximity to other clinics and administrative offices with whom your clients may visit.

ALLOWING FOR GROWTH

The ASLP environment is integrally related to its system of planned growth and expansion. The planning of circulation within the ASLP clinic, which is by nature subject to future change and renovation, must incorporate relevant growth planning criteria. For example, ASLP may be projected to grow in distinct phases. The architectural solution must accommodate this while allowing for a variety of unplanned changes that are likely to occur. Large audiometric test suites with required utility connections do not lend themselves to relocation unless they are specifically designed to be mobile. On the other hand, office space is flexible and can be designed to accommodate future expansion. Every effort should be made to minimize the disruption of services during all phases of construction. This means that some temporary facilities will likely be used for an interim period until all building and safety codes are implemented. Planning for growth implies expansibility, convertibility, and versatility (Rostenberg, 1986). This can be accomplished in several ways, for example:

■ The expansion of the ASLP clinic's hearing aid program or speech-voice science lab creates the need for additional space to house more equipment (Figure 3–5).

■ If a private practice wants to increase the size of its staff, the clinic must expand by adding additional rooms that will correspond to increases in projected work load. For example, two office/speech-language pathology rooms and an additional 60 net square feet for a waiting area might be added for two additional staff members.

■ An existing space can be converted to accommodate a variety of floor plans using a wall partition. This arrangement is flexible enough to accommodate a variety of administrative activities unique to its environment (Putsep, 1974).

■ Space used for multifunctional clinical activities (e.g., stroke clubs, group hearing aid users, office operations) can be versatile enough to accommodate a variety of activities, either simultaneously or sequentially. Some activities, such as office automations, requiring similar equipment can be easily combined.

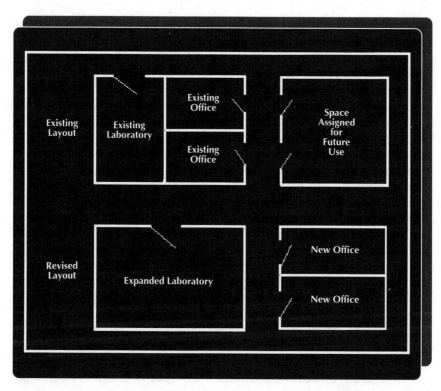

Figure 3–5. Expansion of existing and revised laboratory layout. (Adapted from: Bill Rostenberg Design Planning for Freestanding Ambulatory Care Facilities: A Primer for Health Care Providers and Architects.)

Undoubtedly, space selection may ultimately help dictate whether single versus double-wall constructed audiometric sound suites will be installed. If the room is too noisy for single-wall, then double-wall should be used. Ideally, a newly constructed ASLP clinic should be located at ground level with the prefabricated rooms usually assembled in a floor pit. When audiometric sound suites are installed above ground level, their floor load on the suspended floor joists must be considered in order to be in compliance with federal, state, and local building codes. Double-wall audiometric sound suites should be ordered with the doors piggy-backed, otherwise, an in-swing/out-swing door assembly will be installed by the manufacturer. This creates a problem for clinicians handling nonambulatory patients (e.g., those in wheelchairs or on bed gurneys) when space is limited. In the case of the audiologist who is extremely tall, modifications of the interior height of sound suites must be considered. A detailed treatment of audiometric test room specifications including their total construction, electrical components, ventilation, noise reduction/sound absorption and installation can be found elsewhere (Acoustic Systems, 1991). Examples of the design of neurodiagnostic rooms is presented by Reilly (1987).

An evaluation of existing heating, ventilating, and air conditioning systems should be conducted by an architect or engineering firm to assure year round comfort control and dehumidification. These systems should be designed using parameters specific to the geographic region of the ASLP clinic taking into account the average summer and winter temperatures. Similarly, the electrical system should be evaluated to assure the delivery of appropriate quantities of power. In some older electrical systems the wiring is inadequate to carry the needed currents; this could easily result in a fire safety hazard. In some areas, if the voltage is too low, a waste of energy dollars will occur. In some areas, 60-cycle line noise is a problem. In this case, the support of the engineering department in the hospital is necessary to try to eliminate this artifact. If such service is unavailable, it becomes necessary to avoid electrophysiological recordings in a particular room or area. Even when such areas have been identified, electrical artifact can be variable from day to day. This usually becomes a problem when evaluating patients at bedside. The inability to record at one location does not preclude the possibility that an adequate recording can be made in the same area on a different day or time. Another option may be to use battery-powered equipment.

Sound isolation between rooms is highly desirable in order to eliminate leaks from adjacent areas. A minimum sound transmission class (STC) of 40 dBA (Crocker & Kessler, 1981) should be achieved through construction of partitions with drywall on both sides of metal studs, with two sound attenuation blankets between the studs. The partitions should extend above the ceilings and to the underside of the floor slab above. Penetrations for electrical boxes, lighting fixtures, air conditioning ducts, and grills should be caulked and insulated. Only doors with mechanical seals should be used. Sound attenuation in air conditioning ducts is highly recommended. A sound-absorbent ceiling will prevent sound waves from ricocheting in all directions. Carpet will further reduce noise (especially foot noise), since it absorbs about 10 times more sound than other floor surfaces (Crocker & Kessler). However, carpet becomes a problem for clinicians who have to push moveable equipment around, or move patients in wheelchairs or on litters. This concern can be minimized if low, dense pile commercial carpet is glued directly to the concrete slab rather than installed over pads (Malkin, 1982). When selecting carpet, consideration should also be given to floor surfaces which have been treated for static electricity (which can have a detrimental effect on digital equipment).

The color patterns and furnishings selected for the clinic may be used to accentuate the work environment (Bennet, 1977). The waiting area should utilize soothing colors such as earth tone brown, green, gold, and light shades of blue. Clinical and administrative areas can be decorated in brighter colors such as green and yellow, while avoiding colors such as red and purple. Artwork and murals may also be used to highlight the decor. If the ASLP clinic expects to treat a large number of children, then furniture designed for children to lounge, lie on, or play in has a definite advantage (Lacy, 1979; Malkin, 1982).

The new ASLP clinic should use a mixture of direct and indirect lighting designed to either highlight or de-emphasize certain work areas (Kaufman, 1981; Malkin, 1982). The selection of lighting patterns will significantly contain the cost for electricity if reduced power usage is attained. Since light sources create heat, they will increase the air conditioning systems consumption of energy. Lighting in staff offices and test rooms should contain recessed fluorescent fixtures with external remote ballasts and dimmer switches. Neurodiagnostic rooms should be equipped with recessed incandescent lights to eliminate electrical interference which will contaminate the measurement of electrophysiological events.

After the final clinic design has been selected, the details of the layout must be recorded by an architect. The ASLP administrator and the architect should coordinate their efforts in designing the clinic layout. If modifications to the original design are required, they can be made with consideration of their impact on the clinic's operation. This approach is used by the architect to develop an understanding of the needs and desires of the staff and to incorporate federal, state, and local building and fire codes into the final layout.

EQUIPMENT SELECTION

The scope of services offered will determine the selection of equipment to be purchased. Decisions must be made concerning whether equipment should be purchased or leased (Hampton, 1986). Equipment selection should be based upon past experience, needed requirements, cost(s), reliability, service maintenance, equipment vendor, patient volume, and future expectations. Equipment selection should consist of the following steps:

■ Determine what the equipment is expected to do.
■ Identify, evaluate, and compare similar units of equipment.
■ Select the equipment that meets the expectations of the staff.
■ Prepare a budget for equipment and supplies.

Equipment specification brochures and price quotations should be obtained directly from the manufacturer or its regional representative. Manufacturers must provide technical data to support their product claims. Careful review of their literature will assist in eliminating unacceptable equipment. Other programs using similar equipment should be contacted to provide direct evidence of their level of user satisfaction. The top three manufacturers should be required to provide on-site demonstration of their equipment to evaluate its performance. The equipment should then be prioritized on the basis of user satisfaction and cost to the clinic or hospital.

In federal and state-operated facilities, the purchasing of equipment is the primary responsibility of the purchasing department in the organization. If purchasing obligations were decentralized to each department in the organization, serious management problems would result. Manufacturers would become confused with respect to who in fact has the authority to purchase (buy). The cost for supplies and equipment would escalate because no single control point exists. Legal complications may ensue if manufacturers react to informal, yet implied, agreements instead of formal purchasing requisitions. The integrity of the department and organization may be compromised by allegations of conflicts of interest or unethical business practices. The purchasing process begins with the program administrator who prepares a formal justification that defines the equipment specifications. Competition between manufacturers is essential if optimum cost benefit is to be achieved and if equal opportunity is to be maintained. Requests for purchase of equipment from a specific manufacturer require substantial written justification that said manufacturer is the sole source for a given device. The purchasing department may elect to impose a sealed bid procedure. This procedure is required for purchases of hospital construction or other expensive items (e.g., electrophysiological or speech/voice science equipment).

The selection of the manufacturers to participate in the bidding process is usually based on specific equipment requirements and a comprehensive analysis of all quotations. The purchasing department and the ASLP administrator will determine the cost-benefit of each unit of equipment. Once the final manufacturer has been selected, the purchasing department will complete the agreement between the organization (buyer) and the manufacturer (seller) with a legally binding contract. Most purchasing departments have standardized purchase order forms and contract documents that outline general terms and conditions. For those individuals who are employed in private health care organizations, private universities, or private practices, the choice and outright purchase of equipment may be their own decision to make.

PREVENTIVE MAINTENANCE

Preventive maintenance refers to the performance of nonfunctional repairs, replacement parts, cleaning, and general service to prevent improper and/or inadequate operation, thus reducing down time and extending the service life of the instrument (Carr & Brown, 1981). This is unrelated to calibration which estimates an instrument's performance against standards developed by the appropriate standards institute (e.g., the National Bureau of Standards, Carr & Brown, 1981).

When the manufacturer's warranty expires for each unit of equipment, preventive maintenance becomes the responsibility of the department. Most health care organizations have biomedical repair departments on the premises. Otherwise, the service must be obtained through contractual arrangements. Manufacturers may offer preventive maintenance contracts, but their annual cost may be prohibitive to many clinics. Each unit of equipment should be assigned a unique serial number that is placed on its chassis. This will facilitate the tracking of its maintenance history. Preventive maintenance is usually performed semiannually. The occurrence and duration of unit downtime should also be recorded. All equipment is normally assigned a life expectancy (in years). As this deadline approaches, a decision can be made to either keep the unit in operation or replace it. The Plant, Technology, and Safety Management Standards (Joint Commission on Accreditation of Healthcare Organizations, 1993) provides a format for developing an effective preventive maintenance program to be included in the departmental policy and procedures manual.

CONCLUSION

The ASLP clinic planning and design process is a continuous sequence of activities. The information developed to construct or renovate a clinic should be continually reviewed and modified as conditions change. The ingenuity, persistence, and experience of the program administrator will have a significant impact upon the quality of the final clinic layout. The need to maintain quality service under severe economic pressure is perhaps the greatest challenge facing both the ASLP administrator and architect/designer with whom they will work. The ability to provide affordable services without sacrificing quality of care will determine whether we win or lose in the communication health care business.

REFERENCES

Acoustic Systems, Inc. (1991). Specifications for examination rooms and suites. Austin, TX.

Allen, R. W., & von Karolyi, I. (1976). *Hospital planning handbook.* New York: John Wiley & Sons.

American Hospital Association. (1979). *Signs and graphics for health care facilities.* Chicago, IL: Author.

Bennet, C. (1977). *Human Factor in Design.* Englewood Cliffs, NJ: Prentice Hall.

Berman, H. J., Weeks, L. E., & Kukla, S. F. (1990). *The financial management of hospitals.* Ann Arbor, MI: Health Administration Press.

Carpman, C. J., Grant, M. A., & Simmons, D. A. (1986). *Design that cares: Planning health facilities for patients and visitors.* Chicago, IL: American Hospital Publishing.

Carr, J. J., & Brown, J. M. (1981). Preventative maintenance programs to reduce electrical hazards. In J. J. Carr & J. M. Brown (Eds.), In *Introduction to biomedical equipment technology* (pp. 314–315). New York: John Wiley & Sons.

Crocker, M. J., & Kessler, F. M. (1981). *Noise and noise control,* Vol. 2. Boca Raton, FL: CRC Press.

Fein, D. J. (1983). On aging. *Asha, 8,* 25.

Fein, D. J. (1984). Projection of speech and hearing impairments to 2052. *Asha, 11,* 31.

Folis, J., & Hammer, D. (1979). *Architectural signing and graphics*. New York: Watson Guptill.

Halonen, R. J., & Norville, J. L. (1987). Financial considerations for medical staff office buildings. In Snook, I. D., & Ruck, K. M. (Eds.), *Using hospital space profitably* (pp. 221–240). Rockville, MD: Aspen Publishers, Inc.

Hampton, D. (1986). Establishing and equipping an audiology private practice. In K. G. Butler (Ed.), *Prospering in private practice* (pp 135–147). Rockville, MD: Aspen Publishers, Inc.

Hayward, C. (1985). *A generic process for projecting health care space needs: Committee on architecture for health*. Washington, DC: American Institute of Architects.

Joint Commission on Accreditation of Health Care Organizations. (1993). *Accreditation manual for hospitals*. Chicago, IL: Author.

Kaufman, J. E. (1981). *The IES lighting handbook: 1981 Applications Volume*. New York: Illuminating Engineering Society.

Lacy, M. (1979). Design and planning: A complex process. *Psychiatry Opinion, 16*, 19–26.

Lifton, J., & Hardy, O. B. (1982). *Site selection for health care facilities*. Chicago, IL: American Hospital Publishing.

Lightle, M. A. (1985). Overview of capital financing techniques. In Pena, J. J., & Glesnes-Anderson, V. A. (Eds.), *Hospital management* (pp. 73–83). Rockville, MD: Aspen Publishers, Inc.

Malkin, J. (1982). *The design of medical and dental facilities*. New York: Van Nostrand Reinhold.

Marriotti, J. J. (1982). Office layout. In Gavriel Salvendy (Ed.), *Handbook of industrial engineering* (Chapter 10.6, 1–20). New York: John Wiley & Sons.

Nosse, L. J., & Friberg, D.G. (1991). *Management principles for physical therapists*. Baltimore, MD: Williams & Wilkins.

O'Brien, J. P. (1985). Tax implications for nonprofit hospitals: Unrelated business income. In Pena, J. J., & Glesnes-Anderson, V. A. (Eds.), *Hospital management* (pp. 100–107). Rockville, MD: Aspen Publishers, Inc.

Passini, R. (1977). A study of spatial problem-solving with implications for physical design, Unpublished doctoral dissertation, Pennsylvania State University. University Park, PA.

Putsep, E. (1974). *Modern hospital*. London, England: Lloyd-Luke Ltd.

Reilly, E. L. (1987). *The EEG laboratory: Patient-technician interaction, design, and management* (pp. 86–89). Baltimore, MD.: Urban & Schwarzenberg, Inc.

Reizenstein, J. E., Grant, M. A., & Vaitkus, M. A. (1981). Visitor activities and schematic design preferences (unpublished research report No. 4). Office of Hospital Planning, Research & Development, University of Michigan. Ann Arbor: MI.

Rostenberg, B. (1986). *Design planning for freestanding ambulatory care facilities: A primer for health care providers and architects*. Chicago, IL: American Hospital Publishing.

Schmenner, R. W. (1979). Look beyond the obvious in plant location. *Harvard Business Review, 57*, 126–132.

Snook, I. D., & Ruck, K. M. (1987). *Using hospital space profitably*. Rockville, MD: Aspen Publishers, Inc.

Tompkins, J. A. (1982). *Facilities planning*. New York: John Wiley & Sons.

Veterans Administration. (1980). *Audiology and Speech Pathology Programs* (Chapter 204). Office of Construction. Washington, DC: Author.

Wechsler, S. (1979). Perceiving the visual message. In Pollet, D., & Haskel, P. (Eds.), *Sign systems for libraries*. New York: R. R. Bowker Company.

Recommended Readings

U.S. Bureau of Census. (1983). *America in transition: An aging society*. Current Population Reports (Series P-23, No. 128). Washington, DC: Author.

DeMarle, D. J., & Shillito, M. L. (1982). Value engineering. In G. Salvendy (Ed.), *Handbook of industrial engineering* (sections 7.3.1–7.3.20). New York: John Wiley & Sons.

Francis, R. L., & White, J. A. (1974). *Facilities layout and location: An analytical approach*. Englewood Cliffs, NJ: Prentice Hall.

Harrel, G. D., & Fors, M. F. (1987). Planning evolution in hospital management. *Health Care Management Review, 12*, 9–22.

Jones, H., & Twiss, B. C. (1978). *Forecasting technology for planning decisions*, (pp. 103–111). New York: Petrocilli Books.

Kropf, R., & Greenberg, J. A. (1984). *Strategic analysis for hospital management*, (pp. 7–9). Rockville, MD: Aspen Publishers, Inc.

Pegels, C. C., & Rodgers, K. A. (1988). *Strategic management of hospitals and health care facilities*, XIV, (pp. 24–25). Rockville, MD: Aspen Publishers, Inc.

Posavac, E. J., & Carey, R. G. (1985). *Program evaluation: Methods and case studies*, (pp. 1–29). Englewood Cliffs, NJ: Prentice-Hall.

4

HUMAN RESOURCE MANAGEMENT

Cheryl L. Welch, MBA and Kevin N. Fowler, MS

*"The worst sin towards our fellow creatures is not to hate them,
but to be indifferent to them: that's the essence of inhumanity."*

(George Bernard Shaw, The Devil's Disciple, Act II)

The importance of *human resource management* (HRM) is attracting increasing attention in all facets of health care. Without exception, the success of any enterprise depends essentially upon the effectiveness of the work force, and that effectiveness depends, in turn, upon mutual interests, confidence, and respect. For this reason, ASLP administrators working in programs, however limited or extensive in scope, cannot succeed without the priceless ingredient of good employees.

The program administrator holds the key to successful staff performance. Almost every working day, administrators, managers, and supervisors face some situation related to HRM (e.g., low morale, on-the-job injuries, employee confrontations, staffing shortages, turnover both planned and unexpected, absenteeism, grievances, inadequate performance, compensation, etc.). As the communication link between the staff and senior-level management, the program administrator must set the tone for the department and provide an environment conducive to maximizing staff productivity, thus ensuring the effectiveness and efficiency of the department. To achieve an effective working environment, ASLP administrators must bring to their subordinates an integrated HRM system. The administrator's efforts will have an impact on both internal and external environments as well as on the roles and responsibilities of staff members in meeting the challenges imposed by changing demographics, the economy, state-of-the-art technology, regulatory agencies, and knowledge.

This chapter will concentrate on some of the major HRM issues confronting supervisory personnel and will create an awareness of an increasingly complex area of management. The integrated role that HRM has in the overall effectiveness and efficiency of an ASLP department in today's extremely competitive market will be demonstrated.

PHILOSOPHY AND PURPOSE OF HUMAN RESOURCE MANAGEMENT

A well-defined HRM system is a necessity for a successful ASLP practice. *HRM is the process of formulating the specific personnel mission of the department and making decisions to achieve that mission* (Sethi & Schuler, 1989). In recent years, concepts involving the Joint Commission on Accreditation of Healthcare Organizations (JCAHO), quality assurance, and quality improvement (QI) have promulgated changes in the focus of health care practice, from position descriptions to integrated systems. ASLP administrators are challenged to set high standards of clinical practice and to develop and implement techniques to achieve these standards.

An integrated HRM system relies heavily on establishing a clear set of personnel indicators that guide the ASLP department in analyzing existing and future positions, writing position descriptions, providing recruitment assistance, developing staff, conducting performance evaluations, and providing career opportunities. An integrated approach between HRM and the ASLP department will go a long way toward ensuring that the ASLP department has an appropriate mix of personnel to effectively meet the communication health care needs of each patient.

Sethi and Schuler tell us that an effective HRM system attempts to accomplish the following objectives:

■ Direct the future of a department and its management to minimize the effects of external and internal conditions that affect the department.

■ Incorporate the department HRM plan into the overall organizational plan.

- Create the basis for employee career opportunities.
- Support equal employment opportunity (EEO) laws and affirmative action programs in identifying more diversified populations.
- Reduce personnel cost by recruiting and retaining employees by anticipating shortages before imbalances undermine the program.
- Be cognizant of the impact of technology on the staff in the delivery of health care systems.
- Develop alternate HRM strategies, if warranted.

A systematic HRM plan for the ASLP department must describe the type of work to be accomplished at every level within the department. The ASLP administrator should establish this plan prior to filling the first position.

STAFF ROLES AND RESPONSIBILITIES

Regulatory agencies require that ASLP services be provided by clinicians qualified to meet the health care needs of communicatively impaired patients. Therefore, each position within the ASLP department must be clearly defined and consistent with organizational goals. The ASLP organizational chart should depict the line/staff distribution of administrative, clinical, and clerical positions. However, the question of how each position is analyzed, described, and advertised is critical to the department's success in ensuring maximum productivity, effectiveness, economy, and efficiency. Several essential elements of effective HRM include:

- Review of the ASLP department's structure to avoid duplication of work.
- Determination of the minimum number of positions required to accomplish the department's mission with consideration given to job design, equipment, space, work procedures, methods, and techniques.
- Determination of the mix of personnel (administrative, professional, and clerical) needed and the appropriate compensation for each position.
- Determination of appropriate staff orientation, continuing education requirements, and career advancement opportunities.

Developing a successful HRM strategy to address the above issues does not necessarily require extensive HRM experience. However, the administrator must utilize a design that incorporates job matching by following the hiring process from employee orientation, through job clarification and goal setting, to performance appraisal (Scott, 1983).

POSITION ANALYSIS

Position (job) analysis refers to a systematic process by which the important aspects of a position are identified and documented to reflect the management needs of the department (Middlemist, Hitt, & Greer, 1983). Several relevant purposes of position analysis may include preparing position descriptions and specifications, position classification, position design or redesign, recruitment and selection, performance appraisal, employee training, career development, efficiency, safety, work-force planning, legal requirements, and compensation (Schuler, 1984). Two preferred methods used to obtain information for position analysis include:

- Job (position) focused technique: This method includes direct observation, that is, someone with special training goes to another ASLP site to observe and record how the job is performed.
- Person focused technique: This method may require a meeting with subject matter experts who perform the duties of the job and can provide direct insight into what is required.

The end result of position analysis will describe what the individual in the position is expected to do on a regular and recurring basis. Essentially, position analysis will determine what types of knowledge, skills, and abilities the individual must possess to meet the requirements of the position.

POSITION DESCRIPTION

Position descriptions are essential documents for all departments. A position description provides a synopsis of the unique work requirements for each position. Jones (1984) states that a position description should contain:

- A title, location of the job, date and wage category, and job code.
- A position summary of the major activities, nature of the job, and title of immediate supervisor.
- A description of what is to be done, how it is to be done, and why it is done, using statements that describe the major duties that comprise the position.
- A statement that lists the knowledge, skills, and abilities needed to perform the job.
- The minimum qualifications needed to perform the work. Minimum qualifications are a prime consideration for investigation into EEO and should be stated in terms of specific educational level, training, or equivalent experiences according to preestablished standards.
- A job specifications statement that lists the job and conditions of work used to establish job difficulty or worth. Care must be taken to show that the stated education, experience, and skills required for a particular job are truly necessary to avoid accusations of discriminatory practice (Schuler, 1984).

Position descriptions should be as accurate and complete as possible and should be written in the present tense. Each sentence should begin with an active verb and reflect an objective. Unnecessary words and ambiguities should be eliminated to avoid confusion. Position descriptions should reflect assigned work and employee features (Schuler). Position descriptions have several purposes:

■ They allow administrators, supervisors, and employees to collaborate on what the position should entail.
■ They are a useful management tool for position recruitment, retention, redesign, and potential enrichment.
■ They serve as a document to develop valid performance standards.

With some basic understanding anyone can prepare a position description that accurately reflects the major duties and responsibilities of the job. While minor duties may also be described, they should not influence job qualifications or represent significant periods of time for accomplishment. A position description may not encompass every aspect of the job since some duties may not be included in the statement. However, if these duties are performed regularly and have an impact on the primary duties of the position, then the position description should be reviewed for accuracy. *When several ASLPs accomplish similar tasks, then only one position description of that job is necessary. If the complexity of work performed even at the same level is different, then separate position descriptions must be prepared to reflect such differences.*

Position descriptions may be written in a variety of formats. The most common formats are the *narrative* and *point (rating) systems* (Appendix 4A), respectively. Under the narrative system, tasks are grouped together and evaluated. The tasks identified in the written document are compared against a baseline document that the HRM and ASLP departments have prepared as justification for how a particular job will be compensated. A point system is more complex but when understood is very easy to apply. Under a point system, several factors are described, evaluated against an established standard, and subsequently assigned numerical point values. The point values are totaled and compared to a predetermined value which correlates to an established salary for the position. Regardless of what type of system is used it is more important to understand the types of information needed to describe the position accurately. The uniqueness of each ASLP department must be taken into consideration when developing position descriptions.

RECRUITMENT

Recruiting qualified ASLP candidates is an "art" that may be unappreciated by the employer who wants the position filled immediately. Once an opening has occurred, it becomes necessary to find the right candidate to fill that position. Gellatly (1989) tells us that a recruitment strategy should confront answers to the following questions:

■ Can the position be filled from within the ASLP department? If
so, then there is no need to advertise.

■ Will the search encompass the entire United States? If not, what
are the geographic boundaries?

■ What types of recruitment techniques are presently available to
the various departments?

■ Does the program administrator have access to an established
applicant supply file from which ready referrals can be made?

■ Are financial resources available to cover the expense of placing
classified advertisements in newspapers, radio or TV spots, flyers,
trade journals, billboards, employment agencies, and so forth?

■ Can referrals be identified through co-workers, professional organizations, training programs, labor unions, and so forth?

Recruitment is a commitment by the program administrator to
expend valuable resources to attract qualified candidates who will provide clinical services as well as market the department. The image presented by the program recruiter can have an overwhelming impact on
the decision of the prospective candidate to accept or reject employment.
The image must be honest, up front, and realistic. Equally important is
knowing the appropriate time to recruit. For example, the recruitment of
new college graduates to fill entry level positions should not begin in
September, but in March.

Determining what entices individuals to seek employment with a
specific organization is often elusive at best. Some reasons may include
an established pipeline to a particular site, the geographic location, benefits, potential career opportunities, and so on. Nevertheless, each application should be carefully screened to eliminate those individuals who
do not fit the position description. Active recruitment is also affected by
issues related to EEO and Affirmative Action, for example:

■ Title VII of the Civil Rights Act of 1964, as amended by the Equal
Employment Opportunity Act of 1972, is the federal law that prohibits employment discrimination based on race, color, religion,
sex, or national origin. It prohibits sexual harassment when the
person must submit to such activity to be hired, receive a raise, or
be promoted.

■ The Age Discrimination and Employment Act of 1967, as
amended by 29 U.S. Code 621 et.seq. prohibits discrimination
because of age (in practice, this means persons older than 40
years), conditions, and privileges of employment.

■ The Vietnam Era Veterans Readjustment Act of 1974 provides
preference in hiring to military veterans.

■ The Pregnancy Discrimination Act of 1978, amended and clarified
by Title VII of the Civil Rights Act, requires employers to treat

pregnancy and pregnancy-related medical conditions as any other medical disability.

■ Americans with Disabilities Act of 1990 protects the rights and responsibilities of qualified individuals with disabilities. These rights and responsibilities relate to equal employment opportunity. The law affects federal, state, and local governments and is comprehensive in its coverage. Its guidelines are similar to those of the Rehabilitation Act of 1973 regarding reasonable accommodation. It prohibits discrimination of individuals with AIDS, or those that are recovering alcoholics, or have overcome drug problems, as long as the individual can perform the duties of the job and does not pose a threat to others. It is important to note that the employer is required to make reasonable accommodations, provided the accommodations do not create an undue hardship on the organization.

A successful recruitment strategy should produce prospective candidates. Many organizations have their human resource department coordinate the preliminary interview to avoid duplication of effort, ensure compliance with equal opportunity and affirmative action policies and goals, and expedite the recruiting process. Individuals within the ASLP department may initiate the process or participate in seeking qualified candidates; however, the recruitment process must be coordinated by either the human resource department or by the ASLP administrative section. Those individuals that pass the initial screening process then become candidates to be interviewed.

INTERVIEWING

An interview is essentially a conversation. However, the job interview is a very particular kind of conversation, because it is the ASLP administrator's responsibility to hire the right individual who will strengthen the effectiveness of the clinical team. The concepts described below are important tools in all human service professions. The interviewer's challenge is to judge each candidate's qualifications and match them to the needs of the ASLP department. Metzger (1988) notes that most supervisors are not equipped to interview because of their minimal training in interview techniques, or because they perceive interviewing as a distraction. Pell (1969, p. 102) states that an interview has four purposes:

■ To get information.
■ To evaluate the applicant.
■ To give information.
■ To make a friend.

Metzger (1988) offers some key steps to follow to be effective during the employment interview.

■ Know the job well enough to speak intelligently about it. Review the position description, the work environment, and discuss the position with the immediate supervisor (if applicable) to gain insight into its function.

■ If the position is to be vacated, it is appropriate to conduct an exit interview with the individual leaving the position. This will provide insight into the actual responsibilities of the position.

■ State the purpose of the interview and what is to be accomplished.

■ Stay focused on the interview. Know what to look for to eliminate applicants who do not meet the position requirements.

■ Establish an interview routine and follow it with consistency for that particular position.

■ Review each application or resumé well in advance, and again just prior to the interview.

■ Take notes during the interview to obtain a factual record of information on each candidate.

■ Be honest with interviewees, and let them know how many candidates are being considered for that position.

■ Prioritize the candidates upon concluding the interview process and after staff discussion on this matter.

The interview process should elicit information that will ensure that each candidate's response is clear enough to prevent a wandering discussion. The proper selection of questions is the most important tool to open a discussion, to provoke thinking, to obtain participation, to advance, expand, or terminate a discussion. The success of the interview will depend to a large extent on asking the right questions at the right time. What the interview should yield is a visual portrait that cannot be determined from the application, resumé, or written recommendations. Knowing what types of questions to ask, when to ask them, and what they are intended to achieve will keep the discussion on the interview so that all parties participate. The ASLP interviewer should be thoroughly familiar with various styles of questioning and their proper usage. Martin John Yate (1987) points out twelve types of questions that can elicit information during an interview:

■ Close-ended questions: Does not allow individuals the opportunity to expand on their answer, but can be useful on the application form.

■ Open-ended questions: Requires the interviewee to provide detailed responses.

■ Past-performance questions: Focus on specific experiences associated with previous jobs.

■ Negative-balance questions: Elicit counter-balancing information when everything appears too perfect.

- Negative-confirmation questions: Challenges the interviewee by identifying positive/negative character traits versus one-time incidents.
- Reflexive questions: Control the flow of the conversation to avoid delays.
- Mirror questions: Seek to paraphrase the response to induce further conversation.
- Loaded questions: Probes the decision-making ability of the interviewee (e.g., "what if" type questions).
- Half-right questions: Appear as partially correct statements to see how the interviewee responds. The intent here is to identify individuals who are likely to agree with the boss on most issues or who lack the ability to communicate effectively.
- Leading questions: Persuade the interviewee to respond in a particular way she or he thinks the interviewer wants. Leading questions are discouraged, but they may be used to control the interview or to prevent drifting.
- Layering questions: Elicit responses to questions such as who, what, when, where, why, and how to obtain more discrete information.
- Hamburger-helper questions: Extract more information from the candidate.

It is absolutely inappropriate to ask questions which relate, either directly or indirectly, to EEO issues. Questions related to sex, religion, national origin, age, race, marital status, child bearing, handicaps, or partisan political beliefs should never be asked. Otherwise, this could lead to claims of discrimination against the ASLP interviewer who is representing the department and the organization.

The interview should be conducted in privacy. Every effort should be made to reduce interference as much as possible by transferring telephone lines to someone else, post a "do not disturb" sign, or meet for lunch. Distractions are a nuisance that reduces everyone's ability to concentrate on the purpose of the interview. This is unfair to the candidates who may sense that they are not being taken seriously because essential points of discussion have been overlooked.

The interviewers should be familiar with their own style (e.g., intense, jovial, laid back, overly professional, open, friendly, etc.) to project how receptive the candidate will be. What can the interviewer do to set the candidate at ease since being interviewed is stressful? The interviewer is obligated to establish a proper tone that will meet the objective of selecting the most qualified candidate for the position. Techniques should be used that test the applicant's ability to think quickly, assess their personality, and determine on-the-job performance (e.g., review the candidate's previous work history by eliciting specific work examples or by reading the candidate's body language).

There are a few points of etiquette that should be followed upon conducting an interview:

- Never appeared harried or overburdened.
- Always be cordial.
- Always be truthful. If it is obvious that the candidate is not right for the specific position, communicate this directly using diplomacy and provide a statement of rationale. Should the opportunity exist to be considered for other positions, let the candidate know that their resumé or application will be retained for future consideration. Validate all credentials and references and contact past employers. Remember, the purpose of the interview is to decide to hire or not to hire the candidate, and not the candidate's decision to accept or not accept the position.
- Remain sensitive and do not allow personal prejudices to overshadow the interviewer's objectivity.
- The interviewers should conduct the meeting as if they were the interviewee. This approach should provide maximum success.
- Do not hesitate to interview a candidate two or three times.
- Provide each interviewee with an agenda of events prior to visiting the facility.
- Be on time, well-groomed, and dress appropriately.

Interviewing new ASLPs is very different from interviewing experienced clinicians. New graduates may be anxious, insecure, idealistic, and not totally knowledgeable about what to look for in employment. The ASLP interviewer should identify specific actions taken by the department to assist the new graduates during the transition period from student to practitioner. On the other hand, an experienced ASLP can easily identify what is desired in a new position. The ASLP interviewer can easily focus on these areas and how realistically the department is able to meet these requirements; then additional advantages of the department can be described.

The final phase of the interview is used to clarify any questions, to document salary and benefits, and to arrange for further follow-up. Before the interview ends, both the candidate and the ASLP interviewer need to have a clear understanding of the next step. The final impression of the applicant is just as important as the first one.

STAFF ORIENTATION AND DEVELOPMENT

The success of any organization is based, in part, on its commitment to developing its employees. Shea (1985) points out that few matters affect employees more than the way they are first introduced to their job, to the work environment, and their co-workers. If new employees are loaded down with policy and procedures manuals, given sketchy introductions into what they will encounter, left with unanswered questions and curiosity, they are likely to become dissatisfied and leave. It is extremely important that every new employee be provided an excellent, thorough, and well-planned induction and orientation program that:

■ Reinforces the employees' confidence in their ability to cope with a new work assignment.

■ Communicates, in writing, complete and detailed conditions of a person's employment.

■ Informs the person of the rules and regulations surrounding employment.

■ Instills in the employee a feeling of pride in the institution.

Orientation begins by establishing a good rapport between the supervisor and the new employee. The next step is to establish the same good rapport between the worker and the work to be done. According to Metzger (1988), there are several areas of responsibility that fall to the supervisor in the induction of a new employee:

■ Be cordial and be ready to orient the new employee. Review past experience, education, and training. Have a copy of the current position description, list of duties, and responsibilities available for discussion. Have the work environment, equipment, and supplies ready.

■ Welcome the employees and put them at ease. Indicate the supervisor's work relationship to the employee. Inquire about housing, transportation, and parking.

■ Explain the work of the ASLP department (i.e., its organization and function). Indicate the line/staff position of each employee in the department. Explain the relationship of the new employee to that of the others. Explain whom the employee reports to and who, if anyone, reports to the employee.

■ Tour the facility. Locate elevators, rest rooms, water fountains, eating areas, and exercise facilities.

■ Introduce the employee to other unit supervisors and co-workers.

■ Explain organizational and ASLP departmental rules and regulations (e.g., hours of work, punctuality, attendance, lunch and break periods (if any), requests for leave, use of telephone, smoking policy, etc.), and identify where the policies may be found in writing.

■ Assign new employees to a qualified instructor (sponsor), if warranted.

■ Provide safety orientation and stress the importance of working safely. Show the location of emergency telephone numbers, fire alarm boxes, and extinguishers.

■ Explain departmental policies for protecting patient confidentiality, patient rights, and computer security.

■ Evaluate progress of new employees often during the first few days. Encourage questions and answer them fully. Make corrections tactfully, as necessary, and provide encouragement.

An orientation checklist, based on the above outline, is an excellent tool to be used by the new employee and the ASLP supervisor. The checklist can be tailored to meet the specific needs of the ASLP department.

After completing the orientation, the focus changes to staff development. This can be either formal or informal. It may occur in the work environment or at another site (e.g., workshop, conference, university, etc.). Prior to developing an education and training program, the administrator should perform an educational needs assessment that is specific to each employee. A list of topics should be obtained from the staff, along with suggested speakers. By giving high priority to this activity, the administrator will enhance the effort put into the continuing education program. An education and training program that is diversified in scope should cover the following areas:

■ Supervisory development.
■ Improving professional performance.
■ Cross training or retraining, as position requirements change, because of technological advances or departmental restructuring.
■ Revised JCAHO standards and departmental policy and procedural requirements.
■ Job enhancement.
■ Formal educational opportunities.
■ Career development opportunities.

The question of who is responsible for planning, administering, and evaluating staff education within the ASLP department can be best answered within the specific organization. One option is to have the staff education department in large organizations accept this responsibility. This arrangement works well when select individuals can devote sufficient time to this area. A second alternative is to make continuing education the responsibility of the immediate supervisor in that particular ASLP function. The supervisor may act independently, delegate the responsibility to other members in the unit, or arrange for continuing training from outside the department (contingent upon the availability of funds).

The plan must identify what training will be offered, who will receive that training, when and how often the training will be made available, who will be the instructor, where the training will be offered, and the cost. The training course must have clear, measurable objectives with expected outcomes. For example, what should the employee know, or be able to accomplish, upon completing the course? What skill level is the employee expected to have upon completing the course? What knowledge base is the employee bringing in to the course? How can that knowledge base be expanded? Training seminars are most effective when goals, objectives, and methods are predetermined and clarified by follow-up conversations; and the program is evaluated by the participants. This will determine if the desired outcomes were achieved or require periodic follow-up throughout the year by the immediate supervisor. If the outcomes are short term, it may be necessary to determined the cost effectiveness of the training.

PERFORMANCE STANDARDS

According to Boissoneau, Gaulding, and Calvert (1989):

> Employee performance is the perceived level of competence attained by any employee relative to some established standard. Ideally, acceptable performance is the level of performance exhibited by an employee when the employee understands and discharges all job duties and responsibility effectively. (p. 97)

Developing performance standards is the first step toward evaluating the delivery of ASLP services. Glenin (1974), in discussing performance standards, tells us that the standards serve to establish the quality of care to be judged. This judgment may be according to a rating or other data that reflect the conformity of existing practice with the established standards. The standards must be written, regularly reviewed, and well known by the ASLP staff. Performance standards are the logical outcome from conducting position analysis and writing a corresponding position description. They are used to communicate ASLP goals and objectives, establish accountability for their achievement, and serve as a management tool to assess and improve individual performance. By far the great majority of ASLPs are self-disciplined and well motivated in the attainment of their own pursuits, as well as the department's and the public's best interests. The ultimate objective of performance standards is to improve departmental effectiveness through better use of its human resources. A written performance standard is an expressed measure or level of achievement (including knowledge, quality, quantity, timeliness, objectives, or other matters) as established by ASLP management for the duties and responsibilities of a position or group of positions. Performance standards should be developed for the position and not the person. Employee participation is encouraged in establishing performance standards, which need to be objective, job related, clearly communicated, and easily understood. Employee involvement does not mean the ASLP supervisors must relinquish their managerial responsibility for planning and controlling the work in the unit. ASLP supervisors retain the ultimate right to establish performance standards; however, employee involvement promotes cooperation, respect, and better understanding of expectations.

A performance standard should be comprised of a list of elements or statements which contribute toward accomplishing departmental goals and objectives. An element which refers to any component of an employee's job that is of sufficient importance such that performance below the minimum standards established requires remedial action, is considered to be critical. Failure to perform satisfactorily may result in a promotion being denied, or removal of the employee. Such action may be taken without regard to the performance of other elements of the performance standard. As an alternative, the ASLP supervisor may restructure the position or redistribute the work. In this case, new critical elements and performance standards would need to be established for any change in the position description.

When developing performance standards, consideration should be given to the following questions:

- Is the performance observable?
- Is the performance measurable? What is to be measured? How will it be measured? When will it be measured? Who will measure it?
- Will the evaluator be able to distinguish between different performance levels?
- Is the performance achievable? Are there any barriers?
- Does the employee have substantial control over the position and the authority to accomplish the specific tasks?
- Are the expectations reasonable? Can they be accomplished within the evaluation period?
- Is the performance related to key requirements of the position?
- Is there a performance evaluation system already in place to provide adequate tracking for measurement purposes, or must a system be developed? Most organizations have a system in place for periodically evaluating employee job performance which can concurrently define the need for additional training while identifying rewardable work behavior.
- Are the performance standards valid? Are they reliable? Are they flexible?
- Can the performance standards be used to fulfill interim progress checks?
- Do the performance standards measure outcomes?

Several examples of working performance standards for ASLP personnel are shown in Appendix 4B. Once performance standards have been developed, communicated, and a copy provided to the employee, it is the supervisor's responsibility to transmit individual progress to the employee. Performance standards serve as an incentive in motivating employees since ASLP management should use performance evaluations to adjust pay, grant awards, assess training needs, assign work, and determine promotions, demotions, retentions, and terminations. Every position in the ASLP department should have valid performance standards.

PERFORMANCE EVALUATIONS

The overall purpose of a performance evaluation is to provide an objective and systematic approach to making judgments about employee performance (Tanner & Green, 1986; Wiatrowski, 1987). According to Douglas and Bevis (1979), Wiatrowski (1987), and Grose (1989), performance evaluations are used to:

■ Advise the employees of their level of accomplishment in meeting the position description and performance standards.
■ Recognize employees for their accomplishments.
■ Justify salary increases, promotions, transfers, demotions, or terminations.
■ Attempt to improve communication between the supervisor and employee pertaining to the objectives of the job.
■ Examine the group dynamics of staff members toward the goal of quality improvement (QI).
■ Determine if changes in behavior, attitudes, performance, and job knowledge have occurred.
■ Showcase an individual's abilities within the department.
■ Determine future education and training requirements.
■ Test the validity of the personnel recruitment process.
■ Protect the organization from legal accusations of discrimination.

A performance evaluation (a.k.a., performance appraisal) is intended to reaffirm standards and expectations of clinical practice, recognize accomplishments and achievements, and establish direction for future growth and development (Noble, 1989). The more often employees are provided with interim evaluations of their performance, the closer their performances are likely to meet ASLP departmental expectations. Frequent evaluations also avoid the complaint, "How come nobody told me before that it was against policy?" The employee should be able to expect feedback, both positive and negative, during the course of the evaluation (rating) period. It is inappropriate to withhold performance issues from an employee until a formal review is conducted. Poor performance cannot be corrected if it is not shared with the employee. If poor performance exists, the supervisor must document it and share it with the employee immediately. Some performance evaluation systems contain a checklist of ratings based on the elements contained within the performance standard. The overall rating is based on a definition of performance (Figure 4–1). This approach lends itself to a more unified

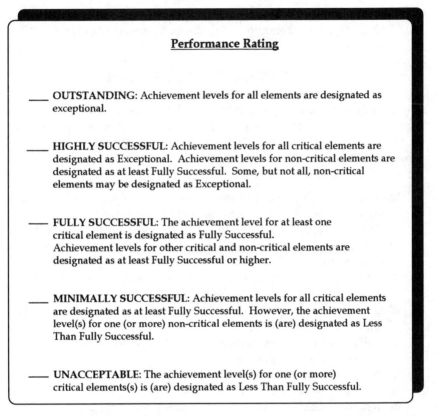

Performance Rating

____ OUTSTANDING: Achievement levels for all elements are designated as exceptional.

____ HIGHLY SUCCESSFUL: Achievement levels for all critical elements are designated as Exceptional. Achievement levels for non-critical elements are designated as at least Fully Successful. Some, but not all, non-critical elements may be designated as Exceptional.

____ FULLY SUCCESSFUL: The achievement level for at least one critical element is designated as Fully Successful. Achievement levels for other critical and non-critical elements are designated as at least Fully Successful or higher.

____ MINIMALLY SUCCESSFUL: Achievement levels for all critical elements are designated as at least Fully Successful. However, the achievement level(s) for one (or more) non-critical elements is (are) designated as Less Than Fully Successful.

____ UNACCEPTABLE: The achievement level(s) for one (or more) critical elements(s) is (are) designated as Less Than Fully Successful.

Figure 4–1. Overall performance rating based on achievement levels assigned to the elements and criteria described in Appendix 4A.

evaluation system among supervisors as compared to using weighted numerical values. For example, some federal agencies use a format which is based on the performance standards that appear in Appendix 4B.

Metzger (1988) notes some pitfalls to avoid when evaluating employee performance:

- Avoid rating employees too high when in fact they may only be average or because of the impact a lower rating may have on career development.
- Avoid being overly critical thereby lowering the overall rating. Raters must have a clear understanding of their own value system, yet be able to demonstrate flexibility.
- Evaluate the performance, not the performer. The best performer may in fact have the most aggressive personality; yet, it is that person's achievement in meeting ASLP goals and objectives that is important. Deal with personality issues separately.

■ Never let an employee's race, religion, sex, national origin, age, marital status, political beliefs, or labor union activities influence the performance appraisal.

If a formal performance evaluation process exists in your organization, it will have clearly defined procedural instructions. Whether you devise your own system, or if there is a preexisting process in effect, do it in privacy. If the workday does not permit this, take the work home.

PERFORMANCE EVALUATION MEETINGS

Performance evaluation meetings require careful planning and preparation to be effective for both the ASLP supervisor and the employee. Prior to the meeting, careful comparison of the employee's performance against the established standards should be accomplished. Employees should include any supporting documents which remind the rater of their accomplishments. This can also reveal ways to improve performance. Employees should present their self-assessment to the evaluator at least one week prior to the conclusion of the evaluation period. Since employees place considerable importance on performance evaluations, every effort should be made to meet during the scheduled time frame. Cancelling and rescheduling performance meetings transmits a negative signal that performance is not important. Performance evaluation meetings should always be conducted in privacy with minimal interruptions. During the meeting the rater should remain focused on the purpose of the meeting. Employees should be allowed to provide their review first. The rater should listen carefully and intervene when it is essential to seek clarification or obtain additional information. The rater should use the same style of questioning applied during the interview process. Remember, the purpose of the meeting is to review past performance and discuss future performance expectations. Metzger (1988) recommends to us that during the appraisal meeting the rater should consider the following:

■ Be sincere, yet specific in evaluating employee performance.
■ Prioritize what is important to develop a written plan to assist the employee in strengthening performance.
■ The written plan should cite any deficiencies, levels of expectation, and should indicate how the employee will receive assistance in meeting these expectations.
■ Additional training should be incorporated into the written plan which identifies who will do the training, where it will occur, when it will occur, and for what period of time.
■ Specify when performance will be reviewed and the consequences of not meeting these expectations. The role of the supervisor is to resolve problems through mutual understanding.

Attention must be given to outside factors that may affect employee performance (e.g., health, emotional, and personal problems, etc.). Although employees may ultimately disagree with their overall rating, they will appreciate the amount of time invested in the assessment if the ASLP supervisor has been thorough and has taken adequate time to explain the evaluation. The meeting becomes productive when future performance expectations can be discussed. No one deliberately wants to perform poorly. An effective meeting should focus on strengths and weaknesses and on the ASLP supervisor's role in assisting the employee to improve professionally. Formal discussions regarding employee performance may occur biannually. However, new employees should have their performance evaluated at three, six, and nine month intervals, and just prior to the conclusion of the first year. Trivial issues should be addressed in another forum because they will distract from the intended direction of the meeting. The appraisal meeting should not reveal any surprises to the employee (i.e., constant feedback during the rating period equals a better understanding of what the meeting will naturally produce).

SUCCESSFUL DISCIPLINE

Every organization has rules and regulations to help employees and management work in harmony with the greatest efficiency. They are designed to make the task of supervising people easier by setting standards so all employees know what is to be expected of them. They provide the ASLP supervisor with authority to keep the department moving ahead with greatest efficiency and minimum friction. The supervisor who is successful in imposing discipline is the person who is capable of getting the work unit to operate smoothly without antagonism and resentment. This requires the supervisor to be prepared to take appropriate action.

Here are some factors (Bureau of Business Practice, 1982) that all supervisors should consider when disciplining an employee:

- Was it an intentional error or something beyond the individual's control?
- What is the past record of the employee? A single infraction is less significant than an established track record in deciding on an appropriate penalty.
- Does the employee have personal problems?
- Was the mistake solely that of the employee, or were others involved?
- What is the work environment?
- Can the employee explain what happened?
- Does the infraction carry a penalty or has it been neglected in the past?

The situation is also influenced by emotions and prejudices. Often, there is not enough time to think through the situation when faced with an immediate problem. It is at this juncture that the supervisor has three alternatives (Bureau of Business Practice, 1982):

∎ Develop an ability to think spontaneously and be able to make a reasonable decision. Discipline employees immediately. Become familiar with their attitudes, work ethics, personalities, and any past disciplinary actions.

∎ Delay making a decision until a determination has been made regarding what happened, why it happened, who is to blame, and whether it could have been avoided.

∎ Prior to the infraction, devise a plan or strategy that applies to the event and all similar events.

Once sufficient information has been obtained to make a sound decision, speak to the appropriate employees in private and discuss your decision and why you made it. Before deciding on the penalty, the supervisor should consider the following?

∎ Does the punishment fit the offense?

∎ Is it covered by established organizational policy?

∎ If the health care organization is unionized, does it violate the terms of the contract? Is it fair, and consistent with past penalties? Is the supervisor prepared to support the decision with documentation if it should be challenged?

∎ What will be the effect on the employee, on obtaining future cooperation if not terminated, and on the morale of the entire department?

∎ Will the supervisor be able to give the employee a clear explanation of the reasons for the punishment? Is the supervisor prepared to explain how to prevent a similar offense in the future?

Certain positions may be covered by a collective bargaining (union) contract and may contain several clauses specific to this issue, such as:

∎ Management must have just and sufficient cause to initiate disciplinary action.

∎ Employees must be treated fairly and equitably.

∎ Discipline must be progressive in nature, unless the action warrants imposing a stiffer penalty.

∎ The action will be taken if it promotes efficiency within the organization.

Progressive discipline refers to initiating lesser penalties for first offenses and progressing through a series of actions that may ultimately culminate in removal. Progressive discipline is designed to correct employee behavior rather than be punitive. Employee misconduct, chronic absenteeism or unauthorized leave, tardiness, abuse of lunch hours or coffee breaks, loafing, drinking alcoholic beverages on the job, dishonesty, failure to comply with ASLP policies and procedures, or any other breach of employee/employer relationship are examples of problems for which disciplinary action may be appropriate. Many organizations have formalized tables of penalties and have guidelines for corrective action. Sample copies of successive letters addressing employee behavior are provided in Appendix 4C. Each successive conference lists preceding actions taken and future actions. Supporting statements, reports, and time sheets should also be attached as necessary. Disciplinary or corrective actions should only be taken to advance the ASLP mission. They should never be taken on the basis of personal animosity or for other prohibited reasons (e.g., discrimination or exercise of appeal). Otherwise, the employee may file a formal grievance (not complaint) against the ASLP supervisor. The human resource department in your organization can provide advice on the appropriate action.

There are four common types of penalties:

■ Verbal reprimand: The process of discussing, in private, an issue that requires immediate attention. For example, an employee has recently established a pattern of reporting to work 10 minutes late. The employee has not demonstrated any past problems. The employee is informed of the issue and what future behavior is expected, and what the consequences may be if immediate improvement is not shown.

■ Written warning: This process formally documents the issue requiring immediate attention. Previous verbal counselings (reprimands) have not resulted in improvement. The written warning is given to the employee, with notification of how long it will be retained in the employee's record, and for what purposes it may be used.

■ Suspension: This action usually involves loss of both money and respect. It is effective but there are disadvantages, such as temporary or permanent loss of the employee through resignation.

■ Discharge: When the attitude of the employee remains poor even after counseling, justification may exist for discharging the employee.

If the ASLP supervisor decides that the only solution to the problem is a suspension, reduction in pay, or removal, compliance with appropriate statutory and regulatory procedures is essential. Previously documented records of progressive discipline will make it easier to initiate adverse action in the event that the collective bargaining employee appeals the decision. Often, too, a record of progressive discipline will support a removal based on the last in a series of minor infractions which by itself would not support removal. It is critical to always keep accurate records to document subsequent, proposed action.

TURNOVER AND RETENTION

Turnover is the nemesis of staffing. Ideally, every organization would like to be fully staffed at all times. Realistically, each organization experiences anticipated and unanticipated turnover for involuntary or voluntary reasons. The key is to minimize unscheduled turnover. This saves valuable man-hour resources in recruiting, training, lost experience, and so forth.

It is important to determine why employees leave the ASLP department since all turnover is not bad. If turnover is linked to conduct issues, a review of policies, guidelines, or regulations may be necessary to determine if they are too restrictive for the work environment. On the other hand, if a poor performer leaves an organization prior to formal action being taken, resources have been saved in the man-hours it would have taken to counsel or prepare formal documents for disciplinary action.

It is equally important for the ASLP administrator to develop a strategy to retain experienced employees. The current labor market for ASLP personnel is so volatile that it has become essential to forgo past employment practices and attitudes regarding senior employees. ASLP departments may participate in local salary surveys to establish creative compensation packages designed to retain long-term employees. For example, employees with more than 10 years of employment might receive an increase in base/hourly pay in addition to any market adjustments, awards, or bonuses to which they may be entitled. Salary, health benefits, rewards, educational training, or career advancement are typical reasons why employees leave an organization. If this is a recurring theme, then the ASLP administrator needs to assess the compensation package. Seldom will disaffected employees cite poor management since they may like the department but not its current financial management philosophy or because they may wish to be considered for future reemployment. When salary is the issue, the ASLP administrator must answer the question, "Is the compensation fair and equitable within the professional community for individuals with like knowledge, skills, and abilities?" If it is not, then the ASLP administrator and his superiors must analyze the cost effectiveness of raising the salary for retention purposes. In the words of Luke (10:8), "For the laborer deserves his wages."

CONCLUSION

The future administrator will be required to be imaginative in the creation of a fully integrated HRM system. Program administrators need to unify employees in developing integrated strategies into a professional culture. This approach will enable the ASLP administrator to cope with the tremendous impact imposed by future knowledge, technology, reimbursement, regulatory agencies, and changing demographics. An unknown author once said, "The best executive is the one who has sense enough to pick people to do what needs to be done, and self-restraint enough to keep from meddling with them while they do it."

REFERENCES

Boissoneau, R., Gaulding, D. J., & Calvert, D. N. (1989). Performance appraisals as a strategic choice for the health care manager. In A. J. Sethi & R. S. Schuler (Eds.), *Human resource management in the health care sector* (p. 97). New York: Quorum Books.

Bureau of Business Practice. (1982). *Training director's handbook.* Waterford, CT: Author.

Douglas, L., & Bevis, E. (1979). *Nursing management and leadership in action* (pp. 198–216). St. Louis, MO: Mosby.

Gellatly, D. L. (1989). Recruitment strategies. In A. J. Sethi & R. S. Schuler (Eds.), *Human resource management in the health care sector* (pp. 75–93). New York: Quorum Books.

Glenin, C. (1974). Formalizing of standards of nursing practice using a nursing model. In J. P. Riehl & C. Roy (Eds.), *Conceptual models for nursing practice* (p. 234–235). New York: Appleton-Century-Crofts.

Grose, L. G. (1989). Choosing a performance appraisal system. In S. M. Glover (Ed.), *Performance evaluations* (pp. 38–46). Baltimore, MD: Williams & Wilkins.

Jones, M. A. (1984). Job descriptions made easy. *Personnel Journal, 63,* 31–34.

Metzger, N. (1988). *The health care supervisor's handbook* (3rd ed.) (pp.108–109). Rockville, MD: Aspen Publications.

Middlemist, R. D., Hitt, M. A., & Greer, C. R. (1983). *Personnel management.* Englewood Cliffs, NJ: Prentice-Hall.

Noble, J. E. (1989). *Making performance appraisal work.* In S. M. Glover (Ed.), Performance evaluations. Baltimore, MD: Williams & Wilkins.

Pell, A. R. (1969). *Recruiting and selecting personnel* (p. 102). New York: Regent Publishing Co., Division of Simon and Schuster.

Schuler, R. S. (1984). *Personnel and human resource management.* St. Paul, MN: West Publishing.

Scott, S. (1983). Finding the "right person." *Personnel Journal, 62,* 894–902.

Sethi, A. S., & Schuler, R. S. (Eds.). (1989). *Human resource management in the health care sector.* New York: Quorum Books.

Shea, G. F. (1985). Introduction and orientation in human resource management and development (p. 591). In W.R. Tracey (Ed.), *Division of American Management Associations.* New York: AMACOM.

Tanner, S., & Greene, L. (1986). Managing the performance evaluation system: A case study. *Health Care Supervisor, 4,* 64–70.

Wiatrowski, M. (1987). Performance appraisal systems in health care administration. *Health Care Management Review, 12,* 71–80.

Yate, M. J. (1987). *A manager's guide to effective interviewing.* Hanover, MA: Adams, Inc.

Recommended Reading

Bureau of National Affairs, Inc. (1992). *Preventing sexual harassment: A fact sheet for employees.* Washington, DC: Author.

APPENDIX 4A

Position Description Narrative Style—Sample 1

JOB TITLE: **Speech-Language Pathologist**
POSITION CODE: _____Salary: _____
DEPARTMENT: Audiology-Speech-Language Pathology
DEPARTMENT HEAD APPROVAL: _____Date: _____
ADMINISTRATIVE APPROVAL: _____Date: _____
DATE OF LAST REVIEW:_____DATE OF NEXT REVIEW: _____

POSITION SUMMARY:

To plan, execute, and control speech-language pathology (SLP) activities, maintain the highest level of clinical standards and good public relations, by creating proactive clinical strategies. Responsible for independent professional action within SLP, subject to general review and consultation with the Department Head. Serves as a member of the professional treatment team, participates in staff discussions of patient diagnoses, progress, and treatment.

PRINCIPAL DUTIES AND RESPONSIBILITIES:

1. Assesses SLP disabilities through the use of diagnostic tests, interviews, case histories, and other appropriate measures. Takes necessary action to effect procedures which will most adequately meet the needs of the patient.
2. Utilizes computer software procedures for electrodiagnostic assessment of the speech motor system, for diagnostic data collection, analysis, and management of a wide range of SLP disorders.
3. Conducts and interprets tests of SLP function to aid the medical community and other specialists in rehabilitative medicine in the diagnosis and treatment of peripheral and central nervous system disorders of the speech mechanism; including expressive and receptive language assessment, right and left hemisphere evaluation, acoustic, aerodynamic, stroboscopic voice analyses, voice rehabilitation, video fluoroscopic evaluation, counsels, provides guidance, and instructs family members on patient care.
4. Develops, with the Department Head, short and long range goals and objectives for a full range of SLP services to be offered; is able to respond to new diagnostic and therapeutic procedures.
5. Is active in developing the SLP quality assurance program, assures compliance with American Speech-Language-Hearing Association (ASHA) and Joint Commission on Accreditation of Healthcare Organizations (JCAHO) standards: maintains an active review

process; identifies problems, plans special studies, and takes corrective action on those problems related to SLP.

6. Ensures that all research conducted in SLP will subscribe to the rules and regulations of the organization for protecting the privacy and safety of the patients or significant others involved in research activities.

LEVEL OF SUPERVISION:
Reports to: Department Head, ASLP
Supervises: Graduate Students

KNOWLEDGE, SKILLS, AND ABILITIES REQUIRED:
Minimum Education:
Masters Degree in SLP (PhD preferred), obtained the Certificate of Clinical Competence in SLP (CCC-SLP), and possesses three to five years of significant clinical experience with neurologically-impaired adult patients; has knowledge in technical and administrative theory and application.

Physical Effort Required:
Ability to walk to the various wards/clinics or sit for long periods of time.

Analytical Skills:
Ability to plan and project future needs in adult SLP; problem-solving skills; good communication within the department and across departments.

WORKING CONDITIONS:
Job Hazard:
May require handling of patients at bedside; may come in contact with patients and personnel with nonsocial infection.

Position Description Narrative Style—Sample 2

JOB TITLE: **Audiologist**
POSITION CODE: _____SALARY: _____
DEPARTMENT: Audiology-Speech-Language Pathology
DEPARTMENT HEAD APPROVAL:_____DATE: _____
ADMINISTRATIVE APPROVAL: _____DATE: _____
DATE OF LAST REVIEW:_____DATE OF NEXT REVIEW: _____

POSITION SUMMARY:

To plan, execute, and control Audiology (AUD) activities, maintain the highest level of clinical standards and good public relations, by creating proactive clinical strategies. Responsible for the independent professional action within AUD, subject to general review and consultation with the Department Head. Serves as a member of the professional treatment team, participates in staff discussions of patient diagnoses, progress, and treatment.

PRINCIPAL DUTIES AND RESPONSIBILITIES:

1. Assesses hearing disabilities through the use of diagnostic tests, interviews, case histories, and other appropriate measures. Takes necessary action to effect procedures which will most adequately meet the needs of the patient.
2. Utilizes computer software procedures for neurodiagnostic assessment of the central nervous system, for diagnostic data collection, analysis, and management.
3. Conducts and interprets tests of auditory function to aid the medical community and other specialists in rehabilitative medicine in the diagnosis and treatment of peripheral and central nervous system disorders of the hearing mechanism, including: puretone air-bone conduction and speech audiometry, acoustic immittance, site of lesion, central tests of auditory processing, tests for pseudohypocusis, electronystagmography (ENG), neurodiagnostic assessment, writes prescriptions for amplification, takes earmold impressions, makes selections, modifications, and responds to the aural rehabilitation needs of adult patients, counsels patients and their family members concerning their hearing handicap.
4. Develops, with the Department Head, short and long range goals and objectives for the full range of AUD services offered; is able to respond to new diagnostic and therapeutic procedures.
5. Is active in developing the AUD quality assurance program, assures compliance with ASHA and JCAHO standards; maintains

an active review process; identifies problems, plans special studies, and takes corrective action on those problems related to AUD.

6. Ensures that all research conducted in AUD will subscribe to the rules and regulations of the organization for protecting the privacy and safety of the patients or significant others involved in research activities.

LEVELS OF SUPERVISION:
Reports to: Department Head, ASLP
Supervises: Graduate Students

KNOWLEDGE, SKILLS, AND ABILITIES REQUIRED:
Minimum Education:
Masters Degree in AUD (PhD preferred), obtained the Certificate of Clinical Competence in Audiology (CCC-A), and possesses three to five years of significant clinical experience with hearing-impaired adult patients; has knowledge in technical and administrative theory and application.

Physical Effort Required:
Ability to walk to the various wards/clinics or sit for long periods of time.

Analytical Skills:
Ability to plan and project the needs of hearing-impaired adults; problem-solving skills; good communication within the department and across departments.

WORKING CONDITIONS:
Job Hazard:
May require handling of patients at bedside; may come in contact with patients and personnel with nonsocial infection.

Point (Rating) System—Sample 3

JOB TITLE: **Speech-Language Pathologist**
POSITION CODE: _____SALARY:_____
DEPARTMENT: Audiology-Speech-Language Pathology
DEPARTMENT HEAD APPROVAL:_____DATE:_____
ADMINISTRATIVE APPROVAL: _____DATE:_____
DATE OF LAST REVIEW: _____DATE OF NEXT REVIEW: _____

Factor 1. Knowledge and ability to administer the duties of an SLP independently including all reports and supervision of graduate students. Ability to communicate effectively orally and in writing will assure the highest probability of success.

SUPERIOR..5

Substantial experience for this position which requires: (a) leadership, management, and supervisory skills needed to oversee the daily operation of the SLP section; (b) building an effective working relationship with the Department Head; (c) oral and written communications, and group dynamic skills to work effectively with students, professional staff, adult groups, and the public. Incumbent will hold a PhD or MA/MS, CCC-SLP, and be eligible for state licensure.

AVERAGE 3

Has some experience in overseeing clinic operations.

MINIMUM 1

Knowledge of administrative techniques with minimal experience in implementation.

Factor 2. Knowledge and ability to assess speech-language disabilities through the use of diagnostic tests and other appropriate procedures to aid the neurologist, otolaryngologist, physician, and other specialists in the diagnosis and treatment of specific speech disorders. Ability to develop group outpatient programs, motivate patients, and interact with families and other professionals.

SUPERIOR 5

Substantial experience for this position which requires: (a) considerable knowledge of assessment and therapeutic techniques for neurologically-impaired adults; (b) supervisory, interpersonal communications, and group dynamic skills to work effectively with students, professional staff, adult groups, and family members. Incumbent will hold a PhD or MA/MS, CCC-SLP, and/or be eligible for state licensure.

AVERAGE 3

Experience for this position would require considerable knowledge of assessment and therapeutic techniques for neurologically impaired adults and some knowledge of supervisory techniques.

MINIMUM 1

Clinical experience in SLP with no actual supervisory preparation.

Factor 3. Knowledge and ability to utilize and develop computer software procedures for diagnostic data collection, management, analysis, and assessment of the speech-motor system. Ability to operate a contemporary speech, voice, and language science laboratory. Interpret measurements obtained from instrumentation such as the visipitch, digital speech spectrograph, laryngograph, phonatory function analyzer, various nonverbal communication devices, language masters and video recording equipment.

SUPERIOR..5

Substantial experience for this position which requires: (a) developing and using commercially available clinical and administrative software in patient care automation; (b) using word processing, electronic spreadsheets, graphics, and data base for administrative, clinical, and research applications; and (c) using speech and voice physiology equipment and integrating their use for clinical research laboratory application. Incumbent will hold a PhD or MA/MS, CCC-SLP, and/or be eligible for state licensure.

AVERAGE..3

Experience for this position would require considerable knowledge of computer and laboratory instrumentation for assessment, therapy, and database management.

MINIMUM 1

Academic (or continuing education) preparation in contemporary instrumentation or computer technology with no actual experience.

Factor 4. Knowledge and ability to develop short and long range goals and objectives for the full range of SLP services offered.

SUPERIOR 5

Substantial experience for this position which requires: (a) selecting and developing goals for the SLP section to respond to the changes of a dynamic communication health care delivery system; (b) effective communication between the incumbent and the Department Head.

AVERAGE 3

Experience in this position would require considerable knowledge of contemporary goals and objectives that affect adult communication disorders.

MINIMUM 1

Academic (or continuing education) preparation in contemporary SLP.

Factor 5. Knowledge and ability to monitor the SLP section's quality assurance program, assure compliance with ASHA and JCAHO standards established by external monitoring groups.

SUPERIOR 5

Substantial experience for this position which requires: (a) developing QA indicators mandated by JCAHO and other regulatory agencies; (b) close scrutiny of clinical activity and appropriate documentation to be in line with the Quality Assurance prerequisites.

AVERAGE 3

Experience in this position would require considerable knowledge of QA/QI goals and objectives that affect adult communication disorders and that are consonant with JCAHO and other regulatory agencies' requirements.

MINIMUM...1

Academic (or continuing education) preparation in contemporary SLP.

TOTAL POINTS ....__

Point (Rating) System—Sample 4

JOB TITLE: **Audiologist**
POSITION CODE: _____SALARY _____
DEPARTMENT: Audiology-Speech-Language Pathology
DEPARTMENT HEAD APPROVAL:_____DATE: _____
ADMINISTRATIVE APPROVAL: _____DATE: _____
DATE OF LAST REVIEW:_____DATE OF NEXT REVIEW:_____

Factor 1. Knowledge and ability to administer the duties of an AUD independently including all reports and supervision of graduate students. Ability to communicate effectively orally and in writing will assure the highest probability of success.

SUPERIOR 5

Substantial experience for this position which requires: (a) leadership, management, and supervisory skills needed to oversee the daily operation of the AUD section; (b) building an effective working relationship with the Department Head; (c) oral and written communications, and group dynamic skills to work effectively with students, professional staff, adult groups, and the public. Incumbent will hold a PhD or MA/MS, CCC-A, and be eligible for state licensure.

AVERAGE 3

Has some experience in overseeing clinic operations.

MINIMUM..1

Knowledge of administrative techniques with minimal experience.

Factor 2. Knowledge and ability to assess hearing disabilities through the use of diagnostic tests and other appropriate procedures to aid the medical community and other specialists in the diagnosis and treatment of specific hearing disorders. Ability to develop group outpatient programs, motivate patients, and interact with families and other professionals.

SUPERIOR..5

Substantial experience for this position which requires: (a) considerable knowledge of assessment and therapeutic techniques for hearing-impaired patients; (b) supervisory, interpersonal communications, and group dynamic skills to work effectively with students, professional staff, adult groups, and family members. Incumbent will hold a PhD or MA/MS, CCC-A, and be eligible for state licensure.

AVERAGE 3

Experience for this position would require considerable knowledge of assessment and therapeutic techniques for hearing-impaired adults and some knowledge of supervisory techniques.

MINIMUM 1

Clinical experience in AUD with no actual supervisory preparation.

Factor 3. Knowledge and ability to utilize and develop computer software procedure for diagnostic data collection, management, analysis, and assessment of the auditory system. Ability to operate a contemporary hearing science laboratory.

SUPERIOR 5

Substantial experience for this position which requires: (a) developing and using commercially available clinical and administrative software in patient care automation; (b) using word processing, electronic spreadsheets, graphics, and data base for administrative, clinical, and research applications; (c) using calibration equipment and integrating their use for clinical research laboratory application. Incumbent will hold a PhD or MA/MS, CCC-A, and be eligible for state licensure.

AVERAGE..3

Experience in this position would require considerable knowledge of computer and laboratory instrumentation for assessment, calibration, and database management.

MINIMUM 1

Academic (or continuing education) preparation in contemporary instrumentation or computer technology with no actual experience.

Factor 4. Knowledge and ability to develop short-and-long range goals and objectives for the full range of AUD services offered.

SUPERIOR..5

Substantial experience for this position which requires: (a) selecting and developing goals for the AUD section to respond to the changes of a dynamic health care delivery system; (b) effective communication between the incumbent and the Department Head.

AVERAGE..3

Experience in this position would require considerable knowledge of contemporary goals and objectives that affect adult hearing disorders.

MINIMUM..1

Academic (or continuing education) preparation in contemporary AUD.

Factor 5. Knowledge and ability to monitor the AUD section's quality assurance program, assure compliance with ASHA and JCAHO standards established by external monitoring groups.

SUPERIOR 5

Substantial experience for this position which requires: (a) developing QA indicators mandated by JCAHO and other regulatory agencies; (b) close scrutiny of clinical activity and appropriate documentation to be in line with the QA/QI prerequisites.

AVERAGE..3

Experience for this position would require considerable knowledge of QA/QI goals and objectives that affect adult communication disorders and that are consonant with JCAHO and other regulatory agencies requirements.

MINIMUM..1

Academic (or continuing education) preparation in contemporary AUD.

TOTAL POINTS ....____

APPENDIX 4B

Performance Standards—Sample 1

Speech-Language Pathologist

These sample performance standards demonstrate the desired expectations to be considered fully successful toward meeting departmental goals and objectives.

ELEMENT

1. **Professional & Technical Services:** (CRITICAL ELEMENT)

   STANDARD:

   1.1 Provides assessment and direct therapy to patients in compliance with appropriate SLP protocols.

   1.2 Daily hours earned for direct services is at least 6 hr spent in direct service activities (assessments, preparing test reports, individual/group therapy, counseling, interdisciplinary meeting, rounds, and screenings).

   1.3 Behaves in accordance with ethical, professional, and procedural standards promulgated by ASHA, state, and regulatory agencies.

2. **Documentation in the Medical Records:** (CRITICAL ELEMENT)

   STANDARD:

   2.1 SLP data bases and test reports are prepared or updated according to SLP content and time standards of an equitable number of assigned patients.

   2.2 There is a clear flow of documentation of clinical objectives and plans from SLP assessments and progress notes according to ASLP department standards.

3. **Proper Use of Instruments, Equipment, and Materials:**

   STANDARD:

   3.1 Evaluates routine and special diagnostic equipment on a timely and accurate basis, and ensures that the equipment and instruments are in proper repair for immediate use with minimal intervention.

   3.2 Applies proper knowledge, methods, and techniques in using specific equipment for testing patients.

   3.3 Inspects, makes minor repairs and adjustments on equipment used in SLP.

4. **Administrative Matters:**

STANDARD:

4.1 Contributes to the process of interdisciplinary functioning by attending special program meetings, as well as scheduled interdisciplinary team and committee meetings.

4.2 Interprets both oral and written instructions received by the Department Head and others.

4.3 Verbal and written reports required, special program and other assignments are accurate, understandable, and complete.

4.4 Completes required reports in a timely and accurate manner to meet time constraints.

5. **Dealing with Others, Habits, Safety, and Risk Management:**

STANDARD:

5.1 Effective in dealing with the Department Head and others. Maintains a positive, professional, working relationship and displays a mature, courteous approach and response at all times in personal contacts.

5.2 Handles routine situations and occasionally refers the more difficult situations to the supervisor.

5.3 Responds promptly to work assignments and other duties such as scheduled meetings, training activities, or special project assignments.

5.4 Stays productive throughout the work day and advises the supervisor of unexpected or unusual delays which would have a significant impact on patient care.

6. **Professional Activities:**

STANDARD:

6.1 Monitors the quality assurance program on a monthly basis; corrects and documents all deficiencies in the appropriate QA folder maintained in the ASLP Department.

6.2 Maintains a cooperative and effective relationship with other service providers, patients, families, and management.

6.3 Maintains and upgrades professional knowledge and skills by completing 20–40 hr of continuing education (contingent upon funding) during the rating period. This will consist of a minimum of 10 hr acquired through formal courses, workshop, seminars, lectures, conferences, and other programs approved by ASHA or affiliated university graduate programs. The balance may be composed of attendance at programs not meeting the above qualifications (e.g., on-the-job training or self-instruction).

7. Computer Information Systems Responsibility

STANDARD:

7.1 Adheres to all regulations and policy guidelines relative to accountability and designated access to all computer information systems.

Performance Standards—Sample 2

Audiologist

ELEMENT

1. **Professional/Technical Services:** (CRITICAL ELEMENT)

   STANDARD:

   1.1 Provides assessment to patients as evidenced by compliance with AUD protocols.

   1.2 Maintains an average of at least 6 hr of on duty time in direct service activities (assessments, preparing test reports, counseling, team meetings, rounds, and, screenings).

   1.3 Behaves in accordance with ethical, professional, and procedural standards promulgated by ASHA and state and federal regulatory agencies.

2. **Documentation in the Medical Records:** (CRITICAL ELEMENT)

   STANDARD:

   2.1 AUD data bases and test reports are prepared or updated according to content and time standards for an equitable number of assigned patients.

   2.2 There is a clear flow of documentation of clinical objectives and plans from AUD assessments and progress notes according to ASLP Department standards.

3. **Proper Use of Instruments, Equipment, and Materials:**

   STANDARD:

   3.1 Evaluates routine and special diagnostics equipment on a timely and accurate basis, and ensures that the equipment and instruments are in proper repair for immediate use with minimal intervention from the supervisor.

   3.2 Applies proper knowledge, methods, and techniques in using specific equipment for testing patients.

   3.3 Inspects, makes minor repairs and adjustment on equipment.

4. **Administrative Communication Matters:**

   STANDARD:

   4.1 Contribute to the process of interdisciplinary functioning by attending special program meetings, as well as scheduled team and committee meetings.

   4.2 Interprets both oral and written instructions received by the Department Head and others.

   4.3 Verbal and written reports, as well as special programs, and assignments are accurate, understandable, and complete.

4.4 Completes reports in a timely and accurate manner to meet time constraints.

5. **Dealing With Others, Habits, Safety, and Risk Management:**

STANDARD:

5.1 Effective in dealing with the Department Head and others. Maintains a positive, professional relationship and displays a mature, courteous approach and response at all times in personal contacts.

5.2 Handles routine situations and only occasionally refers the more difficult situations to the supervisor.

5.3 Responds promptly to work assignments and other duties such as scheduled meetings, training activities, or special project assignments.

5.4 Maintains self productivity throughout the work day and advises the supervisor of unexpected or unusual delays which would have a significant impact on patient care.

6. **Professional Activities:**

STANDARD:

6.1 Monitors the quality assurance program on a monthly basis; corrects and documents all deficiencies in the appropriate QA folder maintained in the ASLP department.

6.2 Maintains a cooperative and effective relationship with other service providers, patients, families, and top management.

6.3 Upgrades professional knowledge and skills by completing 20–40 hr of continuing education (contingent upon funding) during the rating period. This will consist of a minimum of 10 hr acquired through formal courses, seminars, workshops, conferences, and other programs approved by the ASHA. The balance may be composed of attendance at programs not meeting the above qualifications (e.g., on-the-job training or self-instruction).

7. **Computer Information Systems Responsibility:**

STANDARD:

7.1 Adheres to all regulations and policy guidelines relative to accountability and designated access to all computer information systems.

APPENDIX 4C

Written Warning—Sample 1

Date:

From:

Subj:　First written warning to discuss with _____his/her record of being late.

To:

On (date), you were verbally counseled regarding your repeated tardiness in reporting for work as scheduled. Since that date, you have been late on 4 separate occasions (specify dates and include copies of time cards). In each instance, you were informed that your reason(s) for being late were unacceptable. This is to notify you formally that future instances of tardiness will result in you being charged absent without official leave. You will not receive pay for those period(s) of tardiness. It is expected that you will report to work as scheduled, and that you will be ready, willing, and able to perform your job. Failure to demonstrate improvement in reporting to work in a timely manner will result in further disciplinary action being taken.

If you have an alcohol, drug abuse, or biopsychological problem, (e.g., physical, personal, emotional, financial, marital, familial, legal, or job related problem) that is affecting your performance or conduct on the job, you should contact our Employee Assistance program which offers counseling and referral as appropriate for guidance on resolving your problem(s).

A copy of this written counseling will be retained for a period of 6 months, at which time it will be returned to you for your disposal, if it is not used to support an additional disciplinary action because of continued infraction.

_____　　_____

Counselee　　　　　　　　　　　　Date

_____

SUPERVISOR'S SIGNATURE

Note:　It is important that each employee be made aware of, and referred to, Employee Assistance. Trained counselors within the organization, or contracted through a mental health group, can assist employees in dealing with stress, drug and alcohol abuse, and other problems.

Written Reprimand—Sample 2

Date:
From:
Subj: Written reprimand to discuss with _____failure
         to improve his/her record of being late for work.
To:

On (date) and (date), you were scheduled to work from 8:00 a.m. to 4:30 p.m. You reported for work late (specify exact times and include copies of time cards) and are being charged with being absent without official leave for a total of 4 hr for the dates cited. Your conduct in this matter is in direct violation of organization policy (number), which states, " . . . ." Your unauthorized absence(s) have adversely affected the effectiveness and efficiency of your unit in providing essential clinical services to the department.

Failure to improve your timeliness in reporting for work may result in your being placed in a probationary status for further review of your continued employment, or may result in further administrative action being initiated, up to and including discharge.

A copy of this reprimand will be placed in your official employment file. You may, if you wish, make a written reply in explanation of your conduct. If you do, it will also be placed in your official employment file. This reprimand will remain in your file for two years or it may be withdrawn and destroyed after 6 months, depending entirely on your future behavior and attitude. I feel confident that you will earn the privilege of its early withdrawal and strongly encourage you to strive for that goal.

If you believe this action is unwarranted, you may appeal it under the terms of the collective bargaining agreement.

_____   _____
Counselee   Date

_____
SUPERVISOR'S SIGNATURE

Letter Of Termination—Sample 3

Name:
From:
Subj: To discuss with_____his/her failure to improve
his/her record of being late for work.
To:

On (date) and (date), you were scheduled to work from 8:00
a.m. to 4:30 p.m. You reported for work late and are charged
with being absent without official leave for a total of 2 hr for the
dates cited. On (date), an initial written warning was given to
you. A reprimand was written on (date) for additional episodes
of tardiness. Your unauthorized absence(s) have adversely
affected the effectiveness and efficiency of your unit in providing essential ASLP services to the department.

You were placed on 3 months probation from (date) to (date)
and were late twice during that period. Since you have been
unable to correct this problem, I recommend termination.

_____   _____
Counselee   Date

_____
SUPERVISOR'S SIGNATURE

5

QUALITY IMPROVEMENT

Stephen R. Rizzo, Jr., PhD and
Robert T. Frame, DMD, MS

"If you don't keep doing it better, your competition will."

Quality plays a part in the success of every organization. In ASLP, quality begins with the patient (client), the center of clinical focus. To provide quality, all employees from the ASLP administrator down must believe in their program's intention to share vision, mission, and sustain quality of patient care.

PHILOSOPHY OF QUALITY IMPROVEMENT (QI)

In recent years, a long-standing, successful, and more scientific approach to managing quality has surfaced in the health care environment. It is defined in the work of W. Edwards Deming, PhD, a statistician. During World War II, Deming taught the military industry how to use statistical tools to improve the quality of its production (Walton, 1986). After the war, American industry focused its interest on manufacturing consumer goods. Significant foreign competition would not exist for almost another 20 years. While managerial practices were costly, they had little impact on profitability since there was no major competition from outside the United States. At a time when products manufactured in Japan meant inferior quality, Deming was invited by Japanese industrialists to help revive their trade. The Japanese also invited several Americans, most noticeably Peter F. Drucker (author of *The New Society: The Anatomy of Industrial Order*). The Japanese learned that organizations exist to enable ordinary people to do extraordinary things. To accomplish this, the Japanese instilled routine into their daily duties and procedures until their duties became the primary focus of attention. Drucker instilled in the Japanese that the difference between the ordinary and the extraordinary became the extra.

The Deming Management Method (Walton) became known as total quality management (TQM), continuous quality improvement (CQI) or quality improvement (QI). This process has evolved today into a way of doing business affecting every aspect of health care. Leiman's (1992) depiction of this concept encompasses every level of an organization, from senior to middle management, to support services, and direct patient care providers (Figure 5–1). For example, the periphery of the target represents administrative functions, which independently are more process oriented and consistent with TQM. As we approach the center of the target, the emphasis is on the continuous improvement (CI) of patient care. Clinical indicators represent the process that defines the activities between the clinician and the patient. The aggregate of the target represents quality improvement (QI). The key lies in:

■ transforming the organization's culture;
■ defining, measuring, and improving performance indicators related to managerial processes and patient expectations (outcomes);
■ creating a work environment that empowers the employee;
■ implementing team-oriented process improvements;
■ reducing hierarchies within the organization; and,
■ using simple statistical tools to identify and eliminate variations that impede existing effectiveness.

This chapter will focus on how the ASLP administrator creates an environment in which people are not afraid to report problems. The authors will demonstrate the integrated role that QI has toward the reduction of variation in quality services. These principles will be applied to ASLP practice for acceptance by regulatory accreditation agencies.

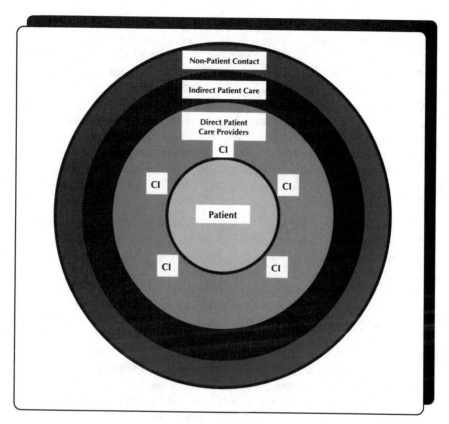

Figure 5–1. The quality improvement (QI) process that encompasses every level of the health care organization. Note: From D. Leiman, DDS, 1992, Kansas City, MO. Reprinted by permission.

IMPLEMENTATION OF QI

QI represents a new way of doing business. It must be customer-focused. The goal is to meet and exceed customer expectations by providing lasting value. Everyone in the ASLP department must be committed to quality. To achieve this, each employee must recognize that each position is a process which can equal efficiency, necessary reevaluations, or rework. This structure must be investigated, measured, analyzed, and improved. The philosophy guides every member of the ASLP department to recognize and be able to monitor significant variations (both inside and outside the organization) that may have an impact on the delivery of clinical services. Processes must be efficient and effective to reduce variation in the way work is performed. Flow charts (to be discussed in the section on the scientific approach) developed by the individuals doing the work are the best starting point. As employees develop flow charts and continue working with them, they will identify and eliminate variation to improving the process. As this variation is reduced or eliminated, employees can better utilize their time.

W. Edwards Deming (1986) and Joseph M. Juran (1987) indicate that at least 80 percent of any individual's failure is the result of the system rather than of the individual. This principle (known as the Pareto Principle) is sometimes called the 80/20 rule and is named after economist Vilfredo Pareto. Juran advises concentration on the fundamental problems and avoiding distraction by those of lesser importance. QI focuses on constant improvement and not on finding fault with individuals. This concept applies to patients, suppliers, vendors, third-party payers, regulatory agencies, and other professional groups. Scholtes (1988) has some recommendations for implementing QI:

- ■ Senior and middle management must lead the transformation effort to ensure lasting success.
- ■ Initiating and implementing a QI strategy will take about two years (others say five years).
- ■ Identify and network people within and outside the department.
- ■ An organization must value its employees in order to retain them.
- ■ Train and educate each employee on QI principles. For example, all employees need to know the relationship between their work and that of the entire department, how it is influenced by workers who precede them, and how their work influences workers who follow.
- ■ Select useful projects for improvement to ensure the greatest success. Projects that are too large or diffuse will frustrate employees and reduce their enthusiasm. Plan the projects in order to assure success.

PROCESSES AND SYSTEMS

The ASLP department is an environment where numerous tasks are performed, such as scheduling appointments; treating patients; calling physicians, school personnel, and vendors; and dealing with third-party payers. QI allows us to look at these tasks as processes. *A process is a sequence of tasks directed at accomplishing a specific outcome.* This may include the sequences in providing a service, hiring a new employee, writing a prescription for a hearing aid, and so forth. Tasks are viewed as a related series of events for each position description (Chapter 4). This will allow each employee to develop an integrated understanding of every position in the ASLP department. For example, how did the appointment get scheduled? Where did the patient come from? How was the patient evaluated? What was the outcome of the evaluation? These processes can be illustrated using flow charting.

A system refers to a group of related processes, such as providing ASLP services. If a team feels overwhelmed by its initial assignment, perhaps it is studying a system instead of a process (Scholtes, 1988). It may be best for the team to narrow the scope of the project, otherwise it may never get off the ground. By way of example, asking the question "How can we improve speech-language pathology testing?" is too broad and does not aid the team in focusing on the details of the process. A better, more specific question might be "How can we reduce the variability in time required to complete an aphasia battery?" This is one way of "setting yourself up" for success.

CUSTOMERS AND SUPPLIERS

Individuals who precede a task are referred to as suppliers, and those who follow the task and receive the service, are customers (Scholtes). External customers purchase products or services. When employees forward their work to other employees, they are internal customers. Similarly, external suppliers are the people outside the ASLP department who provide materials, information, products, or services to the department. For example, when clinicians receive referrals from others in the parent organization, each employee is both a customer and a supplier.

HOW IS QUALITY PERCEIVED?

If customers are the people who benefit from services, only they should determine what quality is to them, what they want, and how they want it. Being able to provide quality products and services at competitive prices requires a reconsideration of what quality is in terms of value and delivery of service. When determining patients' definition of quality, there is one phenomenon that affects the client's (patient's) ability to know quality. A patient cannot always know if the technical quality of the service or treatment they received was the best. They only know how they feel about the care received. This is an area where the peer review process can be used and clinical indicators can be helpful in defining what to measure.

SCIENTIFIC APPROACH

Deming recommends the use of several graphic TQM techniques (or tools) to study, display, and control variations in work processes:

- Flow charts are pictorial representations showing all steps of a work process.
- Fishbone diagrams (or cause-and-effect diagrams) show the relationship between an effect and the possible causes influencing it.
- Pareto charts are a special form of vertical bar graphs that helps to determine which problems to solve and in what order.

■ Run charts are used to represent data visually to monitor a
  process to determine whether the long-range average is changing.
■ Histograms are bar graphs that display the distribution of data,
  or the number of units in each category.
■ Scatter diagrams are pictorial representations of the possible relationship between two variables.
■ Control charts are run charts with statistically determined upper
  and lower control limits, drawn as lines on either side of the
  process average.

Further information on the use of TQM tools can be found in three
publications entitled, *The memory jogger* (Brassard, 1988), *The memory jogger plus+* (Brassard, 1989), and *Tools and methods for the improvement of
quality* (Gitlow, Gitlow, Oppenheim, and Oppenheim, 1989).

Deming points out that the essence of TQM is the scientific approach.
Decisions are based on data rather than assumptions so that managers
respond to the causes of problems and find permanent solutions, rather
than relying on quick fixes. The purpose of using simple statistical tools is
to make it easier to deal with variation.

The following example represents an oversimplification of the scientific approach but attempts to make a point by analogy. Assume the manager determines that 30% of the earmold impressions taken in the hearing
aid laboratory required remake, which signals that a problem may exist. A
flow chart can be used to identify the process to determine if the problem
stems from a technical or procedural error; control charts can be used to
specify cause or systems problem. Both examples address a solution to
correct the problem rather than address the problem as is traditionally
done many times. In short, what can be done to lower the remake rate?
Knowing that a problem exists and doing something about it represent
opposite ends of the spectrum. The basic question is whether the total
number or percentage conceals differences among audiologists. For example, can 30% earmold impression remake be subdivided into groups? The
answer is yes. One basis for subdivision is time of day (Table 5–1)

This subgroup reveals differences in remake rate. Indeed, it appears
all the errors are directly traceable to the night shift. Since the number of
earmold impressions is equal, it is unnecessary to use a weighted average
to arrive at the average remake rate. In this case, we add the remake
rates, and divide by the total number of rates (0% + 0% + 30% = 30%/3 =
10%). By introducing additional subdivisions, and finding significant differences or variation between or among subgroups, the department manager is getting closer to pinpointing the cause of the high remake rate.
Examination of the audiologist's clinical experience working the night
shift reveals a possible explanation for the excessively high remake rate.
It was discovered that all experienced audiologists take earmold impressions during the morning and afternoon tour. It was also revealed that

Table 5–1. Difference in earmold remake rate exhibited by three work shifts.

SHIFT	REMAKE RATE	NUMBER OF EARMOLD IMPRESSIONS TAKEN
8 a.m. to 12 p.m.	0%	100
1 p.m. to 4 p.m.	0%	100
4 p.m. to 8 p.m.	30%	100
		300

only inexperienced audiologists made mistakes. The appropriate data are given in Table 5–2 which indicates that inexperienced audiologists are responsible for errors requiring remake. If the subdivision process stopped at this point, it would appear that more intensive training of inexperienced audiologists could dramatically reduce the remake rate. However, if we introduce one additional basis for subdivision, we may illuminate the cause of the remake problem. What is the composition of the inexperienced audiologist's subgroup? That is, can this subgroup be subdivided on the basis of some characteristic other than the one under investigation? Table 5–3 indicates that audiologists are of two kinds, namely clinicians and student clinicians.

Hence, the process of training student clinicians is the cause of the remake problem. How can the EMI remake rate be reduced or eliminated? A policy can be instituted prohibiting audiology students from making earmold impressions. More careful screening procedures, and more extensive training of student clinicians could be instituted if a no student clinician policy seems too drastic. Either way, remake rate will decline, costs will be lowered, and quality will improve.

Simple statistical procedures can detect significant variations between and among subgroups. Significant variation in the data set might result in further study. The discovery and elimination of variation improve performance. Other processes that can be investigated for variation are:

■ Patient waiting time for appointments;
■ Appropriate communication with patients and families regarding serious communication disorders;
■ Reporting of accurate ASLP test results;
■ The elimination of reevaluations;
■ Scheduling appointments, collection of test results, and report generation; and,
■ Proper maintenance of equipment or test materials.

The key is to improve the quality of each and every performance measurement for the entire staff. There is a need to select appropriate subgroups to detect variation between and among subgroups and to

Table 5–2. Difference in earmold remake rate based on clinical experience level.

CLINICAL EXPERIENCE LEVEL	REMAKE RATE	NUMBER OF EARMOLD IMPRESSIONS TAKEN
Experienced Audiologists	0%	50
Inexperienced Audiologists	0%	50
		100

Table 5–3. Earmold remake problems are caused by student clinicians.

CLINICAL EXPERIENCE LEVEL	REMAKE RATE	NUMBER OF EARMOLD IMPRESSIONS TAKEN
Audiologists	0%	25
Student Clinicians	96%	25
		50

determine if the difference that exists is large enough to indicate that a problem exists.

PROCESS ACTION TEAMS

The projects (issues) selected as important will determine the composition of the process action team. The team members will assume specific responsibilities as determined by their skills and positions within the processes and the organization. Multidepartmental teams are usually self-directed and engage in multifunction problem-solving that crosses several functional boundaries or levels within the organization. These teams:

■ Focus on how to change an organization's thinking about quality improvement, quality control, and quality planning;
■ Detail why project-by-project quality improvement leads to organization-wide quality improvement;
■ Help to define quality;
■ Stabilize a process that has a known capability to produce and is predictable;
■ Communicate that best efforts, intentions, hard work, and experience are not enough to ensure quality;
■ Concentrate on supplier/customer relationships;
■ Collect meaningful data;
■ Demonstrate how quality improvement is continuous and is part of job satisfaction and job ownership by the employees;
■ Help eliminate any resistance when investigating quality of care issues; and,

■ Establish corrective actions for nonclinical processes (e.g., scheduling, billing).

The TQM/QI approach will enable the department manager to achieve dramatic improvements in ASLP practice. Unquestionably, QI is the key to improved health care today. The biggest problems faced by individuals implementing QI are the barriers inherent in organizations run by Management by Objectives (discussed in Chapter 1). People are afraid of giving up their control, or getting involved in something they think could risk their security or position. Acceptance has to be created in the hearts and minds of all. Change happens because people as a group accept it.

Effective teamwork does not happen casually. A systematic process must be learned. An excellent publication on the team building process is *The team handbook* (Scholtes, 1988). This guide is based on the teachings of W. Edwards Deming, PhD. The manual provides information on how to choose team players, work as a team, plan and conduct team meetings, manage logistics and details, and so forth. Team decisions are based on information, not guesswork. Strategies for making team decisions such as brainstorming (a free-form approach to generating ideas), as well as structured approaches to listing options and narrowing them down are discussed.

JOINT COMMISSION ON ACCREDITATION OF HEALTHCARE ORGANIZATIONS (JCAHO)

JCAHO is a private, nonprofit, organization dedicated to improving the quality of care in organized health care settings. The mission statement of the Joint Commission (JCAHO, 1991, p. 3) is:

> The mission of the Joint Commission on Accreditation of Healthcare Organizations is to improve the quality of health care provided to the public. The Joint Commission develops standards of quality in collaboration with health professionals and others and stimulates health care organizations to meet or exceed the standards through accreditation and the teaching of quality improvement concepts.

Initially, JCAHO was considered the watchdog of quality. Health care facilities perceived quality assessment as an obligation, externally activated and governed by fear, to comply with set standards. Today, JCAHO is trying to dispel the notion of forced compliance by shifting to Deming's management philosophy as illustrated in his 14 points (Table 5–4).

Since the mid 1980s the JCAHO has been revising standards on quality assessment and improvement to help healthcare organizations use their commitment, resources, and approaches to improving patient care quality more effectively and efficiently. The JCAHO's *Accreditation manual for hospitals* (1993, p. 139) states "standards place emphasis on the role of the hospital leaders—governance, managerial, medical, nursing,

Table 5–4. Deming's 14 points for total quality management (TQM).

1. **Create constancy of purpose for improving products and services.**
2. **Adopt the new philosopy (i.e., mistakes and negativism are unacceptable).**
3. **Cease dependence on inspection to improve quality. Focus on improvement of work processes and prevention; not inspection after the fact.**
4. **End the practice of awarding business on price alone (e.g., do not adopt a policy of awarding contracts to the lowest bidder). Price has no meaning without an integral consideration for quality.**
5. **Improve constantly and forever every activity to improve quality and productivity and thus to decrease costs.**
6. **Institute training and education on the job.**
7. **Institute leadership and supervision aimed at helping people to do a better job.**
8. **Drive out fear.**
9. **Break down barriers between staff areas. Learn about related departments, what they do, and what problems they have. Work as a team with a common goal.**
10. **Eliminate the use of slogans, exhortations, and targets for the work force unless training and management support are also provided.**
11. **Eliminate work standards that prescribe numerical quotas (e.g., eliminate estimations of quality based on productivity or quantity alone). Quotas take account only of numbers, not quality.**
12. **Remove barriers to pride of workmanship. Assume that everyone wants to do a good job, and don't let bureaucracy, poor supervision, faulty equipment, and outdated methods or procedures stand in the way.**
13. **Institute a vigorous program of education and retraining. The workforce must be educated in new methods, such as teamwork and statistical techniques.**
14. **Put everyone in the organization to work to accomplish this transformation. The commitment must start with top management and be communicated effectively to all levels of the organization.**

Sources: Adapted from *Out of the crisis* by W. E. Deming (1986), Cambridge, MA: Massachusetts Institute of Technology, Center for Advanced Engineering Study; *The Deming management method* by M. Walton (1986), New York, NY: Putnam.

and other clinical leaders—in assessing and improving patient care and emphasize, clarify, and provide greater flexibility in certain steps of the quality assessment and improvement processes." JCAHO has designated this as its "agenda for change."

Currently, ASLP services are surveyed using Physical Rehabilitation Services Standards. Regardless of the type of health care setting the JCAHO (1993) standards manual is designed to be used for continuous self-assessment by the health care organization.

FROM QUALITY ASSESSMENT (QA) TO QI

QA refers to activities performed to assure change in practice that will fulfill the highest level of value. This is accomplished through a ten-step monitoring and evaluation process (to be discussed in the next section). The adoption of QI responds to the need to reduce expenditures for health care services while increasing customer satisfaction. QA will be enhanced with the implementation of QI by incorporating the methodology into a ten-step process familiar to those working in health care settings. The shift from traditional QA to QI has proven effective in many settings. To apply these new principles to everyday practice is important. The use of systematic procedures, effective teamwork, and the application of TQM tools are all prerequisites to managing quality.

JCAHO TEN-STEP MONITORING AND EVALUATION PROCESS

TQM has been incorporated into JCAHO's ten-step process to assess and improve quality. The ten steps below, while directed to health care organizations, in general, have been tailored to meet the needs of ASLPs.

Step 1. *Assign Responsibility*

The organization's leaders (e.g., governing body, chief executive officer, senior management, department heads, direct care providers, etc.) must demonstrate a commitment to QI. These individuals are responsible for implementing and overseeing the process of quality assessment and improvements.

Step 2. *Delineate Scope of Care*

The organization and departmental administrators must identify all key functions. Overall, the scope of care specifies who provides the service (size, type, and qualifications of staff), to whom (patient mix, age groups), what services are provided (e.g., screening, assessment, preventive services, treatment, patient-family education, support groups, and consultation), where services are provided (e.g., onsite, satellite offices, patient's home), and when (e.g., daily, on-call weekend service, hours of service).

Step 3. *Identify Important Aspects of Care*

After delineating the scope of care, the health care organization selects those aspects of care and service that are important to warrant ongoing assessment and improvement. These aspects should be considered most important to the quality of patient care. It is vital to establish priorities instead of attempting to study everything at once. Determining important aspects of care is a process that can be high volume, high risk, or problem prone. For example, hearing aid use processes include prescribing, dispensing, evaluating, monitoring, and system follow-up control. High-volume services affect large numbers of patients, such as hearing screening programs. High-risk services include procedures with potentially serious complications, such as video nasendoscopy or modified barium swallow studies. Problem-prone services (e.g., scheduling conflicts) create problems for staff or patients.

Step 4. *Identify Indicators*

After each important aspect of care is identified, then indicators are selected to measure and monitor the processes or outcome of care. Indicators are a quantitative measure used as guides to monitor and evaluate the quality of important patient-care and support-service activity. They are not a direct measure of quality. They are a signal that identifies or directs attention to specific performance issues that should be topics for further review. Criteria have to be objective and measurable. Process (e.g., ASLP assessments as specified in assessment protocols), or outcome (e.g., early identification of ASLP problems) are important aspects of care for which data are collected in the monitoring and evaluation process.

Clinical indicators can be classified as two general types of events. Sentinel events are incidents which require specific case review (e.g., patient mortality). Rate-based events are linked to the relative frequency and statistical variation which trigger further review of that aspect of care, for example, dysphagia patients who show evidence of subsequent aspiration and receive inappropriate diet and feeding recommendations.

Indicators can also be distinguished by the type of events they measure. *Process indicators measure a patient care activity.* They attempt to measure discrete steps in the patient care process that are important (e.g., conducting audiological evaluations for patients receiving aminoglycosides and loop diuretics whose renal function is at a lower limit of normal). *Outcome indicators measure what happens (or does not happen) to the patient after something is done or not done to the patient.* For example, hearing loss that may result from complications of aminoglycoside treatment.

Finally, the task of developing clinical indicators should involve everyone responsible in that aspect of care. This begins by describing the process using a flow chart. In addition to ASLP-specific QA indicators, the JCAHO (and other external agencies) is interested in indicators that reflect an interdisciplinary team approach to patient care that can be composed of rehabilitation physicians, nurses, clinicians, technicians, and support staff. The team can evaluate clinical indicators as they relate to outcome. QI focuses primarily on the correlation between process and outcome. As you reduce the variation in the process you improve the outcome.

Step 5. *Establish Thresholds for Evaluation*

JCAHO uses the concept of thresholds as a point of reference in the monitoring process. Purists of the Deming school would say that we should "cease our dependence on inspection." Others in the TQM/QI arena may recommend benchmarking. Consistent with JCAHO, each indicator or criterion must have a level, pattern, or trend in data for each indicator that must trigger further evaluation. This is referred to as a threshold, which is frequently a percentage of the extent to which the indicator will be met for the sample number of patients files reviewed. For example, if a 95% threshold is used then 95% of the cases (sample) studied must comply with the indicator. Anything below 95% would trigger an evaluation to determine why the variance has occurred. The 95% threshold allows for 5% variance at one point in time (i.e., it may not stay that way). Once the 95% threshold is reached, the threshold can be raised to strive to improve the quality of care continually or the ASLP can focus on other clinical indicators and aspects of care. Statistical methods (instead of thresholds) can be used to trigger further evaluation.

Step 6. *Collect and Organize Data*

For each indicator, data are collected, analyzed, and compared to the threshold to determine if further evaluation is required. Sources of data can include patient records, diagnostic reports, care plans, progress notes, discharge reports, test scores, survey results, treatment protocol checklists, and staff reports. A data collection process must be designed to answer these questions:

- Who will collect, analyze, and compare the data for evaluation?
- Will data be collected while the patient is being treated (concurrent) or after care has been provided (retrospective)?
- What sampling will be used (e.g., review all cases, review a representative sample of cases, review the first 50 cases)?
- How often will the data be organized and compared with thresholds (e.g., continually, monthly, quarterly)?
- How will the data be displayed (e.g., TQM tools)?
- Can the data be managed by computer technology or will it be handled manually? Computer data base management will streamline the process and increase the efficiency of the activity.

In addition, the data collection mechanism should include a means by which feedback from sources other than ongoing monitoring are used to trigger further evaluation or improvements in other areas.

Step 7. *Evaluation of Care*

A decision is made based on the threshold to determine quality of care. Typically, those individuals who have developed the clinical indicators comprise a team that is ideally suited to evaluate a particular aspect of care. These individuals can represent the ASLP department or interdepartmental processes, if applicable. For example, when a threshold cannot be reached, the team needs to ask two questions:

- What is the reason for the variance?
- How can processes be improved?

The scientific approach, utilizing the TQM tools, can assist in answering these questions. The answer may be found in other tools: department standards, professional expertise, professional association guidelines and standards, and treatment efficacy data published in the professional literature. The goal is to identify work processes that can result in better outcomes. Thus, the focus is on the process and not the provider.

Step 8. *Take Actions to Improve Care*

Once causes and solutions are identified, the proposed actions are implemented. Actions may involve communication channels, departmental procedures, new or replacement equipment, more refined assessment or treatment protocols, as well as adjustments in staffing, changes in chart forms, continuing education, and/or staff assignments. It is here that the staff can be empowered to select and implement changes. The level of empowerment should be defined when the process action team receives its charter from the steering or executive committee.

Step 9. *Assess the Effectiveness of Actions*

Once implemented, actions must be monitored continuously to determine their effectiveness and to sustain improvement. This is the follow-up aspect of QI. Additional monitoring can be initiated at this point. For example, patient satisfaction surveys may provide additional evidence of improved quality. If care is not improved, the team must initiate alternative actions. If care is improved, the team acknowledges this, although ongoing monitoring should continue in order to reflect QI principles.

Step 10. *Communicate Results to Affect Individuals and Groups*

Quality improvements necessitate that the team leader communicates these accomplishments to the appropriate individuals responsible for the work process, as well as to senior level management. Communication is important for maintaining morale, motivation, and employee satisfaction. Reports should specify the findings, conclusions, recommendations, actions, and evaluations of those actions.

For a further discussion of these steps, the reader is referred to the following publications:

- ASHA's guide, *How to establish a quality improvement process: A ten step model* (1992b).

- InterQual, *Quality improvement guide for clinical support departments* (1992).

An example of an ASLP quality assessment and improvement plan appears in Appendix 6A of this chapter.

COMMISSION ON ACCREDITATION OF REHABILITATION FACILITIES (CARF)

CARF is a private, nonprofit organization dedicated to promoting quality services to people with disabilities. Its primary purpose is to identify, through accreditation, those organizations that are rehabilitative in nature and competent in performance. It develops and maintains contemporary standards for use by organizations to measure their level of performance, to promote consumer responsiveness, and to strengthen their programs (CARF, 1992). CARF, since its inception in 1966, has depended on a coalition of national organizations to support the goals of accreditation. Within this coalition, ASHA is a sponsoring member and holds a seat on the CARF Board of Trustees. The CARF Board of Trustees has full authority and responsibility for adopting or modifying standards, awarding or withholding accreditation, and approving basic policies and fiscal matters governing operations.

CARF standards are organized into two sections: organizational standards for the evaluation of programs, physical facilities, health and safety mandates; and program standards for the assessment of the quality of programs for the people served and the comprehensiveness of its rehabilitation programs. According to these standards (pp. 39–40):

- The organization should have an established written system that provides for internal professional review of the quality and appropriateness of the program of services for the person served.
- The review should determine whether:
  - The assessment of the person served was thorough, complete, and timely;
  - The goals and objectives were based on the assessment of the person served;
  - The services provided relate to the goals;
  - The services were provided for an appropriate length of time;
  - The services produced the desired results which are stated in the individual goals of the person served; and
  - The person served has been actively involved in planning and making informed choices regarding the program.

These QI standards require at least quarterly review, and should involve a representative sampling of persons currently served. The review should produce a list of areas needing improvement and actions taken, be integrated into the plan for the person served, and include the results of customer satisfaction surveys. For a review of CARF, as well as JCAHO's survey process for ASLP services, the reader is referred to the work of Cornett (1992).

PROFESSIONAL STANDARDS BOARD (PSB)

ASHA established its PSB in 1959. Its mission is to assure the highest quality of ASLP services, encourage effective clinical management, serve as a recognized accreditation mechanism, and promote quality improvement in-service programs (ASHA, 1989a, p.A-2). Its Council on Professional Standards (Standards Council) develops the standards for accreditation, and the PSB interprets and applies these standards to ASLP service programs.

The PSB evaluates applicant programs and awards accreditation to those operating in compliance with set standards. It also provides the Standards Council with recommendations regarding future standards development. Of particular interest is Standard 25, "Program Evaluation and Quality Assurance." It states, "The program shall evaluate the efficiency and effectiveness of the various components of its operations, including personnel, budget, equipment, facilities, and needs of the population served." The evaluation is accomplished through regular reviews of these components. Such reviews include formal review of individual client management files (p. B-25).

In 1991, ASHA revised this standard in accordance with JCAHO requirements then in place. Implementation was promoted through appropriate and effective patient care and clinical performance utilizing the monitoring and evaluation process. Follow-up activities evaluated the effectiveness of action(s) taken. For example, quality measures follow the same format as described in Joint Commission's Step 4.

PSB is again revising its standards to be consistent with QI methodologies and new JCAHO standards, to be implemented by 1994 (Ulrich, 1991; Anderson, 1992; ASHA, 1992a). The standards will be consolidated and reduced in number from 25 to 8. For example, Standard 3.0, "Quality Improvement Program Evaluation," is designed to monitor and evaluate the quality of services on a continuing basis. Its required characteristics can be found in:

3.1 There are written policies and procedures for evaluating the effectiveness and efficiency of client care and other key areas of program operation.

3.2 Evaluation results are used to improve quality of care and program operation.

3.3 The evaluation process is reviewed and updated on a regular and systematic basis (ASHA, 1992a).

Recently, PSB was encouraged to expand its standards on quality regardless of whether or not a program seeks accreditation.

Accreditation standards, in general, are evolving to reflect the essential beliefs of QI. ASLPs must keep pace with these changes which will occur incrementally over the next several years. It is this yardstick that allows comparison of actual care to a defined "gold standard" to evaluate quality. The *Desk reference (revised)* developed by ASHA (1991) and their *Preferred practice patterns* (March, 1993) specify clinical processes, expected outcomes, and program-specific protocols that may be used as a benchmark against which to measure the quality of care.

MEASURING CUSTOMER SATISFACTION

As QI focuses on the customer, the use of satisfaction surveys is becoming a standard protocol in health care settings. Formerly, the Committee on Quality Assurance (ASHA, 1989b) developed a one-page questionnaire that addressed timeliness of service, physical setting, interactions with staff, and service outcomes. For a more in-depth discussion of this topic, the reader is referred to Chapter 9.

CONCLUSION

The purpose of this chapter was to provide contemporary practices regarding improving quality of ASLP services. The Deming Management Method may be applied to any administrative or clinical work process. However, when all is said and done, this methodology is only part of the picture. We must pay attention to our ASLP profession, be willing to undergo self-examination, and look at our values, attitudes, and behaviors; otherwise no method will be able to thrive. These are strong incentives to change. We may no longer provide ASLP services without knowledge of their cost benefit. To do so would be unethical in light of data-based evaluation of care and limited resources required to obtain adequate reimbursement. The principles of TQM, CQI, and QI afford us the opportunity to acquire new knowledge, can help answer clinical questions, and will help us develop a better way of doing business.

REFERENCES

American Speech-Language-Hearing Association. (1989a). *Professional Services Board: Accreditation standards and manual.* Rockville, MD: Author.

American Speech-Language-Hearing Association. (1989b). *Consumer satisfaction measure.* Rockville, MD: Author.

American Speech-Language-Hearing Association. (1991). *ASHA desk reference (revised).* Rockville, MD: Author.

American Speech-Language-Hearing Association. (1992a). Standards for professional service programs in audiology and speech-language pathology (effective January 1, 1994). *Asha, 34,* 63–70.

American Speech-Language-Hearing Association. (1992b). *How to establish a quality improvement process: A ten-step model.* Rockville, MD: Author.

American Speech-Language-Hearing Association. (March, 1993). *Preferred practice patterns for the professions of speech-language pathology and audiology.* Rockville, MD: Author.

Anderson, C. (1992, Spring). Memorandum re: new charge for the PSB. Supplement to the *Quality Improvement Digest.* Rockville, MD: ASHA.

Brassard, M. (1988). *The memory jogger.* Methuen, MA: GOAL/QPC.

Brassard, M. (1989). *The memory jogger plus+.* Methuen, MA: GOAL/QPC.

Commission on Accreditation of Rehabilitation Facilities. (1992). *Standards manual for organizations serving people with disabilities.* Tucson, AZ: Author.

Cornett, B. S. (1992). Quality and accreditation standards: JCAHO and CARF surveys. *Quality Improvement Digest,* Spring. Rockville, MD: ASHA.

Deming, W. E. (1986). *Out of the crisis.* Cambridge, MA: Massachusetts Institute of Technology, Center for Advanced Engineering Study.

Drucker, P. F. (1950). *The new society: The anatomy of industrial order.* Westport, CT: Quorum Books.

Gitlow, H., Gitlow, S., Oppenheim, A., & Oppenheim, A. (1989). *Tools and methods for the improvement of quality.* Homewood, IL: Irwin.

InterQual (1992). *Quality improvement guide for clinical support departments.* Northampton, NH: Author.

Joint Commission on Accreditation of Healthcare Organizations. (1991). *Transitions: From QA to CQI.* Oakbrook Terrace, IL: Author.

Joint Commission on Accreditation of Healthcare Organizations. (1993). *Accreditation manual for hospitals.* Oakbrook Terrace, IL: Author.

Juran, J. (1987). *Juran on planning for quality.* New York, NY: MacMillan Publishing Co.

Leiman, D. (1992, September). TQI and the development of clinical indicators. Presentation at the Department of Veterans Affairs Clinical Dental Chiefs Meeting, Kansas City, MO.

Scholtes, P. R. (1988). *The team handbook.* Madison, WI: Joiner Associates, Inc.

Ulrich, S. R. (1991). PSB standards, accreditation, and quality improvement. *Quality Improvement Digest,* Spring. Rockville, MD: ASHA.

Walton, M. (1986). *The Deming management method.* New York: Putnam.

Recommended Readings

Block, P. (1988). *The empowered manager: Positive political skills at work.* San Francisco, CA: Jossey-Bass.

Frattali, C. M. (1991). From quality assurance to total quality management. *American Journal of Audiology, 1,* 41–47.

Joint Commission on Accreditation of Healthcare Organizations. (1990). *Committed to quality: An introduction to the Joint Commission on Accreditation of Healthcare Organizations.* Oakbrook Terrace, IL: Author.

Kotter, J. P. (1990). *A force for change: How leadership differs from management.* New York: The Free Press.

Leebov, W., & Ersoz, C. J. (1991). *The health care manager's guide to continuous quality improvement.* Chicago, IL: American Hospital Publishing.

Roberts J. S., & Schyve, P. M. (1990, May). From QA to QI: The views and role of the Joint Commission. *The Quality Letter for Healthcare Leaders.* Rockville, MD: Bader & Associates.

Wender, D. (1990). Quality: A personal perspective. *Asha, 32,* 41–44.

SOURCES OF ADDITIONAL INFORMATION

Periodicals

Quality Review Bulletin (monthly publication).
Joint Commission on Accreditation of Healthcare Organizations.
One Renaissance Boulevard.
Oakbrook Terrace, IL 60181

ASHA's Quality Improvement Digest
American Speech-Language-Hearing Association
Health Services Division
10801 Rockville Pike
Rockville, MD 20852

Hearsay
Journal of the Ohio Speech and Hearing Association
Theme Issue: Quality Improvement in Speech-Language Pathology and
  Audiology
Vol. 7, No. 1, 1992
OSHA Business Secretary
9331 Union Road, South Miamisburg, OH 45342

Journal of Health Care Quality
National Association for Healthcare Quality
5700 Old Orchard Road
First Floor
Skokie, IL 60077-1057

Quality Assurance in Health Care
International Society for Quality Assurance in Health Care
Pergamon Press, Inc.
Maxwell House, Fairview Park
Elmsford, NY 10523

Accreditation Agencies

American Speech-Language-Hearing Association
Professional Standards Board
10801 Rockville Pike
Rockville, MD 20852
(301) 897-5700

Commission on Accreditation of Rehabilitation Facilities (CARF)
101 North Wilmot Road, Suite 500
Tucson, AZ 85711
(602) 748-1212

Joint Commission on Accreditation of Healthcare Organizations
One Renaissance Boulevard
Oakbrook Terrace, IL 60181
(708) 916-560

Professional Associations

National Association for Healthcare Quality
5700 Old Orchard Road
First Floor
Skokie, IL 60077-1057
(708) 966-9392

APPENDIX 6A

QUALITY ASSESSMENT AND IMPROVEMENT PLAN—SAMPLE

The intent of this example is to define the policy, procedures, scope, and assignments of responsibility for an organized and systematic approach to quality management. Stephen R. Rizzo, Jr., PhD, Chief, Audiology & Speech Pathology Service, Department of Veterans Affairs, Chillicothe, Ohio, has contributed this example, along with monitoring and evaluation models.

   I. PURPOSE:

      The ASLP Quality Assessment (QA) Plan provides for the monitoring and evaluation of care delivered to all patients, corrects identified problems, and reevaluates corrective actions. This program is designed to be dynamic and flexible. Changes of indicators and criteria will be made as necessary.

  II. OBJECTIVES OF THE QA PROGRAM:

    A. Establishment of a systematic approach to monitor and evaluate the quality of ASLP care in an ongoing and continuous manner.

    B. Evaluation of patient outcomes to assure quality of patient care.

    C. Establish a systematic process for analyzing and correcting problems and identifying opportunities for improvement.

 III. MONITORING AND EVALUATION MODEL:

    A. Step 1: Identification of Responsibility:

       1. The ASLP administrator has overall responsibility for execution of the QA program and has ultimate responsibility for implementation of corrective actions for identified variances.

       2. The ASLP QA Committee is composed of two audiologists, two speech-language pathologists, and the department secretary. The purpose of this committee is to evaluate trends and recommend actions on items that require a more intensive review, a change in an established program or procedure, or involve additional long term planning. The composition of the QA Committee will be:

               ASLP Administrator
               Staff Audiologists
               Staff Speech Pathologists
               Service Secretary

B. Step 2: Delineation of Scope of Care:
1. The ASLP Service provides comprehensive hearing and speech health care to all referrals in need of treatment. The major diagnoses treated are peripheral (sensory) auditory disorders, otoneurologic disorders of the auditory and vestibular systems, prosthetic management of hearing loss, voice disorders, organic or psychogenic disorders, and disorders of language (aphasia), thought, and memory.
C. Step 3: Important Aspects of Care:
1. Patients undergoing neurodiagnostic recording techniques and interpretation.
2. Hearing aid management.
3. Evaluation and documentation of communication disorders, appropriate therapy, and recommendations.
4. Evaluation and documentation of appropriate speech-language therapy and recommendations in the medical records.
5. Patients undergoing dysphagia evaluation.
D. Step 4: Identification of Indicators and Criteria:
1. See Appendix A.
2. ASLP indicators and criteria will be developed by staff members and presented by the ASLP administrator to the entire staff for approval. Indicators will be forwarded to the medical center's Quality of Care Advisory Board for final approval. The following data and references will be used (along with other available material) in developing the criteria:
   a. current acceptable ASLP standards of care.
   b. staff recommendations
E. Step 5: Establishment of Thresholds for Evaluation:
1. See Appendix A.
2. ASLP staff will establish indicators and criteria for each aspect of care. For each criterion, the staff will establish a threshold level which, when met, will require further intensive evaluation.
F. Step 6: Collection and Organization of Data:
The ASLP Service will monitor and collect data for the purpose of evaluating the quality of care given to eligible patients. Collected data will be presented to the staff for analysis, identification of specific patient care problems, and evaluation of the effectiveness of corrective actions previously implemented by the ASLP Service.
G. Step 7: Evaluation of Care when Thresholds are Reached:
The ASLP administrator will trend the QA Committee's findings and present them to the QA Committee which will

identify problem areas and determine if opportunities to improve patient care exist. Actual outcomes will be compared with expected outcomes. Problematic issues will be reviewed by peers and the results will be reported quarterly or semi-annually at the ASLP Service QA and staff meetings.

H. Step 8: Actions to Improve Care:

The ASLP Service will institute a feedback loop in QA to change or improve the quality of care. In-service educational programs will be held to resolve any problems identified in the QA program. This activity will be documented in the monthly ASLP Service QA meeting minutes, followed by monitoring to assess and maintain improvement.

I. Step 9: Assessment of Action Effectiveness:

The ASLP QA Committee will continue to monitor the identified problems, using the same criteria and data collection processes, after corrective actions have been implemented. To assess sustained resolution of the problem and documentation of the provision of quality care, the monitoring and evaluation process will continue until improvements are noted.

J. Step 10: Communication of Relevant Data:

1. The ASLP QA Committee meeting minutes will be communicated to the ASLP staff at the monthly service staff meeting.

2. These minutes will include findings, conclusions, recommendations, actions taken, and evaluation of actions for committee approval and concurrence by the ASLP administrator. These minutes contain confidential information and will be retained in a secure manner in the ASLP Service for three years.

3. These minutes will be forwarded to senior management through the Medical Center Quality Management Coordinator.

IV. Annual Appraisal:

The ASLP administrator is responsible for analyzing the effectiveness and comprehensiveness of the QA program. The annual program appraisal is due November 1 each year.

Signature, ASLP Administrator

Date

Attachment: Appendix 6A-1

APPENDIX 6A-1

MONITORING AND EVALUATION

Aspect of Care: *Patients undergoing neurodiagnostic recording techniques and interpretation.*
Indicator: Auditory brainstem response evaluations
Type: Problem prone.
Threshold: 90%
Criteria: Yes   No   N/A

   1. Were individual wavepeaks, interpeak, and
      intrapeak comparisons consistent with the
      appropriate recommendations?   ____   ____   ____
   2. Were appropriate recommendations made
      to the treating physician?   ____   ____   ____

Data Source: Medical Record
Sample Size: A representative sample (100%) of auditory brainstem response (ABR) evaluations were performed during a 3 month period.
Methodology: Data will be monitored by the ASLP QA Committee. Patient files, maintained in the service, will be retrieved monthly by the service secretary to assure adequacy of sample size. The data will be collected, analyzed, and compared by the ASLP administrator once per quarter. The findings, conclusions, recommendations, action, and follow-up are discussed with the entire staff at ASLP Service monthly staff meeting, and are documented and sent to management for review.

Approved by members of the ASLP Service at a staff meeting on January 14, 1993.

MONITORING AND EVALUATION

Aspect of Care: *Patients undergoing vestibular recording techniques and interpretation.*
Indicator: Electronystagmography (balance) evaluations
Type: Problem prone.
Threshold: 90%
Criteria: Yes   No   N/A

1. Were tests results consistent with the
   appropriate recommendations?   ____   ____   ____
2. Were appropriate recommendations made
   to the referring physician?   ____   ____   ____

Data Source: Medical Record
Sample Size: A representative sample (100%) of the electronystagmography (balance) examinations were performed during a 3 month period.
Methodology: Data will be monitored by the ASLP QA Committee. Patient files, maintained in the service, will be retrieved monthly by the service secretary to assure adequacy of sample size. The data will be collected, analyzed, and compared by the ASLP administrator once per quarter. The findings, conclusions, recommendations, action, and follow-up are discussed with the entire staff at ASLP Service monthly staff meeting, and are documented and sent to management for review.

Approved by members of the ASLP Service at a staff meeting on January 14, 1993.

MONITORING AND EVALUATION

Aspect of Care: *Hearing aid management.*
Indicator: Patients receiving hearing aids.
Type: Problem prone.
Threshold: 90%
Criteria: Yes   No   N/A

1. Were accurate earmold impressions made?   ____   ____   ____
2. Was there noticeable improvement (in dB) in
   functional hearing, as perceived by the patient? ____   ____   ____
3. Were additional hearing aid adjustments
   requested by the patient to enhance listening? ____   ____   ____

Data Source: Medical Record
Sample Size: A representative sample (100%) of the hearing aid(s) were fitted during a 3 month period.
Methodology: Data will be monitored by the ASLP QA Committee. Patient files, maintained in the service, will be retrieved monthly by the service secretary to assure adequacy of sample size. The data will be collected, analyzed, and compared by the ASLP administrator once per quarter. The findings, conclusions, recommendations, action, and follow-up are discussed with the entire staff at ASLP Service monthly staff meeting, and are documented and sent to management for review.

Approved by members of the ASLP Service at a staff meeting on January 14, 1993.

MONITORING AND EVALUATION

Aspect of Care: *Evaluation and documentation of communication disorders, appropriate therapy, and recommendations.*
Indicator: Patient education.
Type: High volume.
Threshold: 90%
Criteria: Yes   No   N/A

  1. The patient (and significant other)
     understood the diagnostic findings and
     therapeutic goals as they appear in the
     medical records.   ____ ____ ____

Data Source: Medical Record
Sample Size: A representative sample (100%) of patient records were reviewed during a 3 month period.
Methodology: Data will be monitored by the ASLP QA Committee. Patient files, maintained in the service, will be retrieved monthly by the service secretary to assure adequacy of sample size. The data will be collected, analyzed, and compared by the ASLP administrator once per quarter. The findings, conclusions, recommendations, action, and follow-up are discussed with the entire staff at ASLP Service monthly staff meeting, and are documented and sent to management for review.

Approved by the members of the ASLP Service at the staff meeting on January 14, 1993.

MONITORING AND EVALUATION

Aspect of Care: *Evaluation and documentation of appropriate speech-language therapy and recommendations in the medical records.*
Indicator: Aphasia
Type: High volume.
Threshold: 90%
Criteria: Yes   No   N/A

    1. The outcome of therapy is consistent with
       the diagnostic test results.   ____ ____ ____

Data Source: Medical Record
Sample Size: A representative sample (100%) of aphasia patient records were reviewed during a 3 month period.
Methodology: Data will be monitored by the ASLP QA Committee. Patient files, maintained in the service, will be retrieved monthly by the service secretary to assure adequacy of sample size. The data will be collected, analyzed, and compared by the ASLP administrator once per quarter. The findings, conclusions, recommendations, action, and follow-up are discussed with the entire staff at ASLP Service monthly staff meeting, and are documented and sent to management for review.

Approved by the members of the ASLP Service at the staff meeting on January 14, 1993.

MONITORING AND EVALUATION

Aspect of Care: *Patients undergoing dysphagia evaluation.*

Indicator: Patients evaluated videofluroscopically for dysphagia with evidence of subsequent aspiration and appropriate diet and feeding recommendations made to the attending physician.

Type: Rate-based.

Threshold: 100%

Criteria: Yes   No   N/A

1. The outcome of diet and feeding techniques
   do not place a dysphagic patient at risk.   ____ ____ ____

Data Source: Medical Record

Sample Size: A representative sample (100%) of dysphagic patient records were reviewed during a 3 month period.

Methodology: Data will be monitored by the ASLP QA Committee. Patient files, maintained in the service, will be retrieved monthly by the service secretary to assure adequacy of sample size. The data will be collected, analyzed, and compared by the ASLP administrator once per quarter. The findings, conclusions, recommendations, action, and follow-up are discussed with the entire staff at ASLP Service monthly staff meeting, and are documented and sent to management for review.

Approved by the members of the ASLP Service at the staff meeting on January 14, 1993.

6

MANAGING PRODUCTIVITY

John A. Page, MS

"*Don't measure yourself by what you have accomplished, but by what you should have accomplished with your ability.*" (John Wooden, Coach, UCLA)

Individuals affected by communication disorders invest considerable dollars in ASLP services each year. In return for that investment, program administrators are expected to give an accounting of how the money was spent and with what result. Pressure from tightening cost restraints and excessive competition from others occasionally makes the challenge of ASLP management seem impossible. In response to these challenges, program administrators must rise to the occasion, looking for information that will enable them to provide quality care and manage productivity so that their departments can survive. In general, as a department improves the match between staff and workload, the utilization of staff (worker productivity) increases.

To some extent, this chapter picks up where the previous chapter "Quality Improvement" leaves off. The author provides specific examples of how higher productivity can be achieved through the improved management of workload and staffing patterns. This chapter also gives an overview of how to measure workload, determine staffing requirements, and interpret productivity monitoring reports to achieve increased productivity.

WHAT IS PRODUCTIVITY?

Productivity can be described as the relationship between work effort (resources used to produce the output) and physical output used in the production process. In health care, productivity is typically measured in terms such as billed hours per patient day or the amount of time a clinician spends in providing direct patient care. Time is usually referred to in units (e.g., one unit = 15 min).

The goal of any attempt to improve productivity should be to "work smarter, not harder." Simply increasing the rate at which employees operate does not, in the long run, provide substantial increases in productivity. Such an approach to increasing productivity may also cause additional undesirable effects, such as a reduction in the morale of personnel or negative impact on quality of care. These impacts can have disastrous consequences which outweigh any short-term productivity increase that may be achieved. Therefore, a major objective of increasing productivity is to eliminate obstacles that impede effective and efficient operation.

PHYSICAL VERSUS FINANCIAL PRODUCTIVITY

Many factors influence the productivity of any particular group of employees. Included in these are the quantity of resources (i.e, labor and supplies) consumed. For example, productivity of ASLPs (measured in terms of patients seen, procedures performed, and discharges per day) would obviously be significantly influenced by:

- Severity of the communication disorder.
- Age of the patient.
- The skills, motivation, and attitudes of employees.
- Scale of operations (service utilization).
- Organizational work flow.
- Managerial competence.
- Equipment automation.
- Availability of materials, space, and so forth.

Many of these issues have been discussed previously in preceding chapters of this book.

Another factor that significantly affects productivity and is of special importance to the entire health care industry is the quality of service. It is a fairly widespread assumption that high productivity and high quality are mutually exclusive options. For this reason, high productivity (reduced time to perform work) is unattainable, and presumably undesirable, if quality is to be ignored to achieve it. In reality, high quality and productivity can be compatible and both can be accomplished. To achieve this objective, program administrators need to know what quality is in their department and how to manage it effectively and efficiently. Therefore, what is desired is to operate within the range where high productivity is achieved while high quality is maintained. The question that must be answered is, "How can that managed range be achieved?" The challenge to the ASLP administrator is to identify this range and to manage departmental resources within this range.

In as much as physical productivity refers to the efficient use of resources, productivity can also be viewed in terms of the value created. Any business can be highly efficient in providing services, but this does not assure that the output is effective in satisfying customer needs and that it thus has value. Many health care analysts recommend the computation of financial productivity (profitability). This computation is obtained by dividing value added (revenues minus products and services purchased from others) by one or more physical inputs (e.g., labor hours or number of available appointment times).

In the business sector, profitability is generally considered the best overall indicator of company performance. Profitability represents the consequence of managerial decision making (i.e., the products or services produced, marketing strategy, level of investment, and, the efficiency with which inputs are converted to outputs). Since financial productivity is a proportion of dollar value added to dollar (not physical) inputs, the resulting cost-effectiveness ratio is essentially a measure of profitability. Kopelman (1986, p. 5) states it another way,

$$
\begin{aligned}
\text{Profitability} \quad &= \quad \frac{\text{output quantity}}{\text{input quantity}} \times \frac{\text{sales price}}{\text{cost price}} \\[2mm]
&= \quad \text{physical process productivity} \times \text{price recovery} \\[2mm]
&= \quad \frac{\text{output quantity} \times \text{sales price}}{\text{input quantity} \times \text{cost price}} \\[2mm]
&= \quad \frac{\text{revenues}}{\text{expenses}}
\end{aligned}
$$

In essence, physical productivity is a prerequisite but not a sufficient condition for economic success. Everything else being equal, the higher the probability of physical productivity, the greater the likelihood that an enterprise will survive and thrive economically (van Loggerenburg & Cucchiaro, 1981). Although physical productivity does not assure success, certainties are few and far between in any undertaking. Finally, to improve productivity adequate measures of work must be developed and maintained. The importance of physical productivity is discussed, in more detail, in the following sections.

SYSTEMATIC APPROACH TO PRODUCTIVITY IMPROVEMENT

Despite the basic assumption made by many people, productivity improvement is more than just cutting staff. There is no doubt that productivity can be improved by reducing the resources used in producing any given volume of work. However, it can also be improved by doing more with the same resources, less with a proportionately greater reduction in resources used, or more with a proportionately smaller increase in resources consumed.

Today's health care organizations have an increasingly high-profile emphasis on doing "more with less." Hence, program administrators must become unbiased, objective observers who must identify the impact of departmental activities on the entire health care organization they represent. They must identify and develop solutions to operational problems which inhibit high productivity. This logical approach requires a review of departmental operations and the interactions of its components. In industrial/management engineering parlance, this process is referred to as the systems approach and involves the following stepwise actions to uncovering and analyzing operational problems:

- Define the question (e.g., are we appropriately staffed in ASLP?).
- Define the problem (e.g., current expenses in ASLP exceed revenue by several thousand dollars).
- Establish the method for studying the problem.
- Anticipate the results of the study.
- Evaluate the cost-benefit of the study.
- Perform the appropriate study.
- Redefine the problem and solution parameters.
- Define alternatives.
- Test alternatives (feasibility and cost-benefit).
- Present findings.
- Sell alternatives.
- Implement the program.
- Follow up on performance.

Typically, program administrators have a broad range of patient care standards (outcomes), performance standards (employees' responsibility), and resource standards (productivity targets) as the basic area of knowledge from which to draw. Because of the highly interactive and patient-dependent nature of health care, the administrator must also be able to apply traditional analysis techniques to a unique and sometimes more complex set of circumstances.

ACHIEVING HIGHER PRODUCTIVITY

To improve operational efficiency, department managers must understand what is done and how the work is being completed. This can be achieved by discussing departmental operations with the staff on a daily basis. The operation described in a department's policy and procedure manual may not resemble the day-to-day operation of the department. Therefore, it is extremely important to review each process by which work is completed, observing the interaction of personnel and flow of work to understand the true operation. The secondary benefits to be derived from this approach will enhance departmental understanding of recommendations made and the human resource management aspect of supervising people affected by subsequent changes in operation. Several areas that should routinely be considered when trying to increase departmental productivity include a review of the workload, operating budgets, workload scheduling, staffing patterns, fluctuations in workload volume, facility layout, and interdisciplinary relationships:

Review Previous Work Load

A clinical procedure performed by a clinician is considered one unit of work. This value must be easily counted and take approximately the same amount of resources and work hours to complete among providers. The work load of the department represents the total number of units of work projected or actually produced during a given period of time. The ASLP administrator must determine how many units of work load will be performed in a budgeted year and then calculate the amount of personnel resources needed to do the work. For example, if the work load for the past year was 5,000 clinic visits and present marketing efforts should produce a 6% increase in patient volume for the budgeted year, then the work load for the budgeted year is:

Work Load = Work Load for Current Year × (1 + percent increase)
Work Load = 5,000 × 1.06
Work Load = 5,300 patient visits

Work load measures what the department produces or does. It does not measure what the product or services are used for or how it may benefit the patient. It is important to analyze all historical data such as workload volumes on procedures performed to introduce any changes to procedure-patient mix. Remember, given the changing demographic practice patterns, similar procedures performed are not considered equal. While a routine diagnostic examination counts as one procedure performed, the evaluation of a difficult-to-test patient is quite different, in terms of resources consumed and the number of personnel required, when compared to the same procedure performed on a cooperative patient. For this reason another procedural description may be recommended with a different "charge code." Review of historical data can also be used to identify (and quantify as much as possible) past changes and to anticipate future program changes. For example, what impact will an additional otolaryngologist on the ENT staff have on the ASLP work volume? What will the new emphasis on rehabilitation do to the patient mix? By anticipating these changes in advance, increases in productivity can be obtained. Once a predetermined level of productivity is established, the program administrator must be able to answer the question, "What is it going to cost (i.e., labor, supplies, and equipment)?"

Review Operating Budgets

Review of available operating expense data, such as payroll, supplies, equipment, and so forth, can provide significant insight into the clinic operation. Examination of past departmental budgeted and actual hours per procedure can give insight into productivity problems. Historically, hospitals have attempted to solve operational problems by increasing staff positions. However, that luxury can no longer be accommodated. Improving organization-wide labor productivity may require additional dollars to be expended in other clinical departments. All of us can think of an example where being "penny-wise but pound foolish" seemed to be the order of the day. Some additional cost may be required to obtain far greater returns from increased productivity. For example, a department may increase departmental costs by hiring a typist/transcriptionist, but may enhance clinician productivity since reports can be dictated by the clinician rather than typed, allowing the clinician to perform additional procedures.

The importance of cost as a financial indicator is significant. The cost of providing the desired hours per clinic procedure is based on skill level mix, the time it takes to provide care or service at different levels of acuity, and average salary. Cost can be used as: (1) baseline information for determining a profitable price, (2) an indicator of whether current costs are exceeding the current price; and/or, (3) criteria for determining the potential profitability of the department. These uses represent planning functions. Knowledge of labor consumption by specialty function will allow the department to be competitive in the marketplace by offering the customer high quality clinical services. The volume of clinic procedures is used to determine labor requirements and costs. Direct (permanent) staff positions are allocated on the basis of hours per clinic procedure (plus the indirect and nonproductive hours built on top of the direct hours). The precise accounting of total departmental costs paves the way for accurate pricing of services. Analysis of patient acuity data, volume, and financial data helps the ASLP administrator reassess the budget, adjust it, and prepare for the next budget cycle. Monitoring these activities will provide excellent retrospective data for further planning decisions.

In general, budgeting procedures allow the department to expand and contract the budgeted "bottom-line" resources (including labor) based on the actual workload. However, as one might imagine, without accurate and appropriate workload measures and consistent monitoring by management, such a philosophy can be disastrous. For a more in-depth discussion on the topic of financial management, the reader is referred to Chapter 8.

Review Workload Schedules

Work schedules represent the time pattern that employees follow on the job. Work schedules represent one aspect of the use of labor in the productivity process. They are used to match the production needs of the enterprise with the human needs and availabilities of workers. Work schedules vary according to: (1) length of work time (e.g., 40 hr per week), (2) allocation of work time (e.g., 8 or 10 hr per day), and (3) control over work time (e.g., by managers and employees).

Fixed work schedules are usually set by management for most employees and consist of five 8 hr days per week starting at 9 a.m. and ending at 5 p.m. For some individuals, overtime hours may be available as approved by management. Alternatives to traditional work schedules may be available (e.g., using part-time employment as well as changing the standard full-time work schedule to four 10 hr days). Part-time employment options include temporary employment, permanent part-time employment, job sharing, work sharing, phased retirement, sabbaticals, and work year contracts. A predetermined length of work time can be changed by using staggered work hours, flexible work schedules, or compressed work-weeks. The use of flexible work schedules shifts some control over work schedules from managers to employees.

By maximizing the various workload schedules, the administrator can provide significant opportunities for productivity improvement. This can include the use of additional appointment times (5 p.m. to 8 p.m.) to accommodate working adults. These opportunities may allow the administrator to alter marketing strategies and to improve consumer relations through reduction of "over-booked" schedules. Hence, workload leveling can eliminate the peak-and-valley syndrome typically associated with health care services.

A major goal of productivity improvement should be to improve the match between the available personnel resources with the workload to be completed. Particularly within the human service sector, workload often does not fit smoothly into a "9–5" workday. Through innovative and irregular scheduling mechanisms (e.g., split and staggered shifts, part-time personnel, 10 hr 4 day work-weeks, etc.) the ASLP administrator can achieve significant productivity gains. An added incentive to innovative scheduling mechanisms can be improved staff morale. For example, the staff can be scheduled to work four 10-hr day weeks (on a rotating basis) which gives each employee a 3-day weekend at predictable intervals. The interval depends on the size of the staff. ASLP staff hired into budgeted positions are prescheduled according to annual staffing patterns. However, every day there are potential variances from the anticipated, budgeted average. The labor standard (to be discussed in the next section), combined with daily scheduling information, gives the ASLP administrator the information needed to make appropriate staffing decisions.

It is equally important to consider how effectively the department manages staff fringe benefit time or nonproductive time (e.g., continuing education, vacation time, sick leave usage, and daily break time). Significant losses in productivity may be tied to poor management or abuses in the use of employee fringe-benefit time.

Skill Mix

The actual staff-skill mix is an important consideration to understanding how staffing affects productivity. Are the right people routinely available to complete the work? Remember, having the appropriate number of bodies available to perform the workload says little about the ability of those personnel to meet the given volume demand (i.e., have the right people been hired?). A careful review of other descriptive materials (e.g., existing job descriptions, and policy and procedure manuals) can provide additional insight into the ASLP operation to prevent any oversights. For example, does a job description written in 1992 (or 1982) apply to that position today? Typically, managers say that keeping job descriptions updated is a futile and meaningless chore because nobody really reads them. Proactive administrators use job descriptions to define current needs and the necessary levels of staff qualifications. Second, they develop the descriptions with an eye to the future, so that the job descriptions reflect anticipated requirements as well. (For a more in-depth discussion on the topic of human resource management, the reader is referred to Chapter 4.)

Fluctuations in Workload Volume

Many clinical departments follow distinct volume fluctuation patterns. Seasonality, or other fluctuations of activity, leads to department peaks and valleys that will significantly affect productivity. For example, one

ASLP program reviewed was affected significantly by the practice patterns of three otolaryngologists. These physicians were avid clinical researchers who were on leave to attend several professional conferences annually. This practice led to a significant decrease in referrals to the ASLP department (during these times). The department had not adjusted staffing to account for these predictable volume valleys, thus reducing department productivity. Other types of volume fluctuations (e.g., time of day, day of week, monthly, or seasonal variations) can also affect productivity and must be considered.

Facility Layout

Since the facilities area may require a more significant financial investment to correct than other areas mentioned, many ASLP departments are hesitant to deal with problems inherent in the current department layout. Granted that with 20/20 hindsight we can all identify where in the process we should have been concerned with the functionality of any work environment (i.e., the initial planning and design phase of construction). As effective administrators we wish to be proactive, not reactive; ideally, the operation of the ASLP department should be considered prior to the construction phase. In reality, the impact of the facility layout on operations is sometimes underestimated or ignored during planning and layout, eliminating potential productivity improvements, probably forever. We are sometimes overwhelmed by making decisions related to the color of wallpaper or the size of the waiting room, yet fail to consider how the department will actually function after construction. However, given that the ASLP administrator can probably do little to renovate diagnostic and therapy rooms after construction (without significant investment of additional capital), there are modifications that can be made to increase productivity. Some considerations might include the replacement of stationary office desks with movable (modular) workstations. The layout of movable equipment is an important consideration too, and one that may have little or no associated construction costs. A systematic arrangement of the work environment to streamline activity flow and work is essential. (For a more in-depth discussion on facility planning and design, the reader is referred to Chapter 3.)

Interdepartmental Relationships

The delivery of ASLP services does not occur in a vacuum, but requires the interaction of many departments and personnel. Identifying interdepartmental relationships can provide many opportunities for maximizing productivity of the entire organization. Many managers fail to recognize that what occurs in their programs can sometimes affect other departments. This "ripple effect" can be quite significant, and must be considered when proposed changes in operations are made. Although increased coordination of efforts should yield increased staff productivity and improved patient care, fiscal pressure to reduce patient length-of-stay within the health care environment may foster competition among departments rather than cooperation in patient scheduling. Astute managers look for means to reduce the intra-institutional competition.

DEVELOPING LABOR STANDARDS FOR PRODUCTIVITY IMPROVEMENT

To assess utilization of staff and departmental performance, administrators must first develop labor standards. A labor standard is the amount of time (on the average) required by staff to produce a unit of work. Four steps to be followed when developing labor standards (that will ensure reliability and acceptance among departmental personnel) are:

- Identify and define ASLP activities performed in a department.
- Select activities that represent work load indicators being measured (e.g., audiologic evaluations).
- Determine the time required to complete the procedure.
- Determine the frequency of occurrence.

Identifying and Defining the Department's Activities

The first step to developing ASLP labor standards is to identify the activities performed in the department. Labor standards must address both effectiveness (the right thing) and efficiency (the right way). Definitions of what constitutes a process to perform a specific procedure may vary from organization to organization or even between personnel within any given department. Proper and complete identification and documentation (i.e., a procedure description) eliminates the possibility of misinterpreting the data and will improve the interpretation of the data for subsequent review.

Documentation of activities can be accomplished through various methods including narrative descriptions, activities flowcharting, and process charts (for further discussion on this topic, the reader should refer to Chapter 5). Although any method of documentation may be used, a combination of these three can provide a sufficiently detailed record of the activities performed.

As part of the definitions process, a department's activities can be classified into two categories: variable and fixed. Variable activities are those which fluctuate due to changing volumes. Variable activities include routine audiologic examinations, hearing aid evaluations, language, and voice therapy sessions, and so forth. Fixed (or constant) are those activities that are essentially unaffected by fluctuations in patient volumes. These activities might include CPT (current procedural terminology) code checks, performing inventories, administrative meetings, calibration, continuing education, and in-service functions. As one might imagine, these activities are not directly affected by patient volume fluctuations and remain constant, at least within a relative range. This relative range can be illustrated as a step function (Figure 6–1).

Activities within each category may also be classified as direct (patient care activities) or indirect (support activities performed by departmental personnel). Direct variable activities would include procedures performed on patients, whereas indirect variable activities include billing, filing, scheduling, and other activities. ASLP administrators need to take indirect activities into account when the time comes to determine the size of the required staff (to be discussed later in this chapter).

Selecting Workload Indicators

Once the department's activities have been identified and defined, appropriate work load indicators must be selected. These indicators must be quantifiable and must give a good indication of the entire work load within the department. The level of detail necessary may vary from department to department. Some departments may require a significant amount of detail to determine their work load adequately; others can use fewer indicators. It should be understood, however, that the greater the detail desired for measuring work load, the greater the effort will be to develop labor standards and the greater the commitment will be to gather the needed data continually. Direct patient care indicators can be based on the procedure mix (such as with CPT coding categories; air/bone conduction threshold testing, auditory brainstem response, speech, voice, dysphagia evaluations, etc.) to define work load appropriately.

When choosing workload indicators, the ASLP administrator should consider the "80/20 rule" and concentrate on the 20% of department procedures that account for 80% of the volume. It is more important to have good and accurate measures on high-volume activities than to have less-than-accurate measures on all procedures. (For example, a clinic procedure performed once a month in a department would not be as critical an indicator as one performed 10 times per day.) When determining volumes for department activities, program administrators will find that some volume data are more easily obtained than others, such as those that can be provided by the hospital billing system. Variable activities such as ASLP procedures may be utilized as work load indicators.

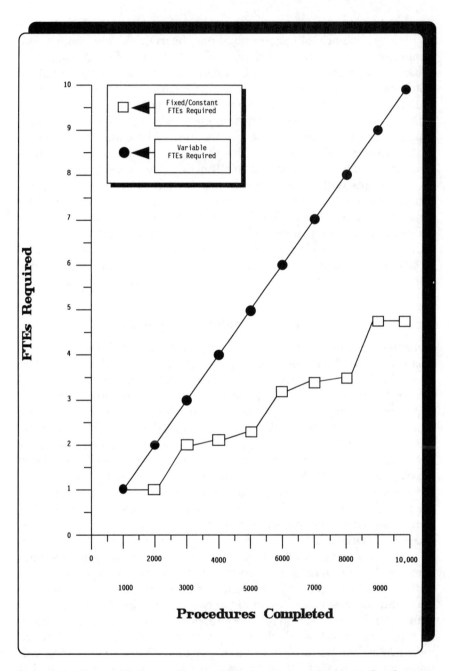

Figure 6–1. Direct and indirect staffing needs. Source: *From productivity and performance management in health care institutions* (1st ed., p. 73) by M.D. McDougal, R.P. Covert, & V. B. Melton, (Eds.), Chicago: American Hospital Association. Reprinted (or Adapted) by permission.

It is not unusual, however, for a ASLP department to think that the charge codes defined in the current billing system do not adequately define the workload within the department. This may be because the charge codes do not adequately differentiate between various procedures with respect to different levels of resources required or because the definitions are unclear or outdated. Here, the ASLP department has the choice of either updating the charge codes or selecting alternate ways of measuring workload and obtaining those values.

Developing Labor Standards

Labor standards provide a detailed and accurate measure of the time required to complete a given procedure in ASLP (Table 6–1). There are several methods for developing labor standards, such as work sampling in which random observations of work are made to estimate the proportion of the workday being spent on various activities. Another is self-reporting/diaries, in which workers themselves are asked to record the amount of time they spend in various tasks. Both of these methods can estimate, over a specified period of time, the total hours utilized for spe-

Table 6–1. Identifying workload indicators and comparison of volume adjusted budgeted procedure hours to actual provided hours

Procedures	*Budgeted Standard Hour/Procedure	× Volume	=	Total Hours Earned	Actual Hours = Staff × 8	Variance ( ) = Under Target
Routine Audiological	1.0	× 50	=	50	47	(3)
Hearing Aid	1.0	× 45	=	45	50	5
Balance (ENG)	1.5	× 38	=	57	53	(4)
Neurodiagnostic(s)	1.0	× 40	=	40	46	6
Aural Rehabilitation	0.5	× 26	=	13	15	2
Language-Cognitive	1.0	× 36	=	36	40	4
Voice-Resonance-Articulation	1.0	× 40	=	40	40	0
Dysphagia	1.0	× 20	=	20	25	5
Totals	8.0	295		301	316	(15)

*These values are for purposes of illustration only. Typical usage may vary, but greater accuracy than one-half hour increments is more common.

cific activities that have been designed as workload indicators. These estimates should include only those hours actually worked. Nonproductive hours, such as those for vacation, holidays, sick leave, and so forth, should not be included.

Once the total hours have been estimated for a particular activity, they are divided by the volume of activity during that specified period of time. The result is an elementary labor "standard." For example, if a department determined that 1,000 hours were worked to perform 800 ASLP evaluations in the past year, the labor standard could be 1.25 hours worked per ASLP evaluation (1,000 divided by 800) taking into account total staff time (i.e., multiple staff members). An alternative to performing calculations such as this is to use preestablished ASLP standards (if available), rather than have the department determine standards for itself.

Another alternative for developing labor standards is participative analysis, which brings staff members of a department together as a group with knowledge of the activities performed in the department. A modification of the Delphi approach (Delbecq, Van de Ven, & Gustafson, 1975; Burack & Mathys, 1979) is used to achieve a consensus on what the labor standards should be. The Delphi approach may be time-consuming but can improve the long-term benefits of productivity by fostering departmental acceptance as well as improving the accuracy of the results obtained.

Whatever approach is used for developing labor standards, administrators must ensure that they are updated as necessary to maintain their integrity. Only labor standards that are accurate can be utilized as a starting point in staffing for productivity improvement. A labor standard that addresses only doing the right thing may provide sufficient time to deliver patient care. However, if the plan for delivery is inefficient, it will have a negative impact on the viability of the department in trying to achieve unrealistic goals. Conversely, if a labor target is incomplete (i.e., it does not include all direct activity to perform the evaluation), it can inhibit an employee's ability to perform the desired level of work.

DETERMINING UTILIZATION TARGETS

Once labor standards have been established for the ASLP workload indicators, the administrator needs to determine a desired target for the utilization of the staff to better manage staff utilization and performance. Established targets (in %) convey the desired match between staff and work load. For example, a department with a utilization target of 90% is expected to have some unproductive staff time (i.e., excess capacity) available to react to uncontrollable or less controllable operational factors (Table 6–2).

Table 6–2. Factors affecting staff utilization.

Controllable Factors	Less Controllable or Uncontrollable Factors
• Scheduling of staff • Easily scheduled work load • Prioritizing work load and postponing deferrable work load to slower periods in shift, day, week, month, and year • Avoidable delays • Scheduling of vacations • Job sharing (intradepartmental and interdepartmental) • Reducing downtime by sending employees home early when work load permits (if policy allowed/required such action)	• Substantial work load fluctuations throughout day, shift, week, month, and year • Unavoidable delays • Physician ordering patterns • Stat orders • Quality of service expectations (e.g., turnaround time and waiting time) • Sick leave • Market constraints regarding the availability and use of part-time positions for improving the match between staff and work load

Source: From *Productivity and performance management in health care institutions* (1st ed., p. 76) by M. D. McDougal, R. P. Covert, & V. B. Melton, (Eds), (1989), Chicago: American Hospital Association. Reprinted by permission.

While identifying (actual) levels of utilization among ASLP management and staff may seem relatively easy, determining an exact utilization target is not. Nonetheless, three methods used to approximate utilization targets are as follows:

■ Review historical (actual) levels of utilization among other clinical departments and negotiate with top management an appropriate utilization target.

■ Quantify all delays and downtime, rectify the avoidable delays, and establish the utilization target on the basis of the unavoidable delays and acceptable levels of downtime (e.g., minimal staffing requirements for providing acceptable levels of service).

■ Calculate an overall weighted-average utilization target on the basis of the distribution of work load by shift and the accepted utilization levels by shift (or portion thereof). This computation is obtained by multiplying the percentages of work load for each shift by the percentages of expected utilization. An example of this method, representing an ASLP department's typical heavy morning work load, is provided in Table 6–3.

Establishing a utilization target for any department quantifies the expected performance of that department by management/administration. Factors specific to particular departments are difficult to generalize. Nevertheless, for overall reference, Table 6–4 provides a listing of a typical department and should be used for overall guidance in establishing utilization targets.

Table 6–3. Weighted average utilization target for an ASLP Department, based on work load fluctuations by shift.

Shift	Percent of Work Load (1)	Expected Utilization (Percent) (2)	Weighted Utilization (1 × 2)
Morning	45	95	0.428
Afternoon	20	65	0.130
Evening	35	75	0.263
Total	100		0.821
Weighted average utilization target 82.1%			

Source: Adapted from *Productivity and performance management in health care institutions* (1st ed., p.77) by M. D. McDougal, R. P. Covert, & V. B. Melton, (Eds.), (1989), Chicago: American Hospital Association

DETERMINING THE SIZE OF THE REQUIRED STAFF

The next step in assessing both utilization of staff and departmental performance is to determine the total number of paid Full-Time Equivalents (FTEs). One FTE represents one year's worth of paid time for one employee (i.e., Hr per FTE = 8 hr × 5 days × 52 weeks = 2,080 hr per FTE). The term FTE has come into use because of part-time employees. The very nature of part-time employment is that these employees do not contribute a full year of work within a calendar year. Therefore, an equivalent in work-years must be used. For example, two half-time employees would equal one FTE (i.e, 2 × 0.5 FTE = 1 FTE). Nonproductive FTEs represent positions/hr budgeted to cover hours that are paid, but not worked. This will vary depending on approved benefits. For example, 15 vacation days + 8 holidays + 6 sick days x 8 hr per work days = 232 annual nonproductive hr per FTE. For example, one FTE would be expected to be "productive" (available to produce workload) 1,848 hours per year (2,080 − 232) and the nonproductive allowance is 12.55% (232 divided by 1,848). In any case, the total FTE is computed as follows:

■ (Add together the volumes for the direct variable activities (work load indicators) to determine the total activities (hereafter referred to as "procedures"). The result is Quantity A. (Table 6–5 provides an example of this and subsequent calculations described in the following steps.)

■ Multiply the volume per procedure over a given period by the labor standard per procedure to determine the standard hours per procedure for that period. Then add all the standard hours together. This sum is the direct procedure hours (Quantity B).

Table 6–4. Typical utilization targets for hospital departments.

Department	Typical Utilization Target
Ancillary Services	
Electrocardiology	80–95%
Electroencephalography	89–95%
Laboratory	80–95%
Pharmacy	80–95%
Physical Therapy	80–95%
Radiology	70–95%
Respiratory Therapy	80–95%
Nursing Services	
Critical Care	75–95%
Emergency Room	60–90%
Labor and Delivery	40–80%
Medical/Surgical Unit	90–100%
Nursery	70–90%
Obstetrics	75–95%
Operating Room	70–95%
Pediatrics	75–95%
Recovery Room	70–90%
Support Services	
Administration	85–100%
Admitting	75–95%
Business Office	90–100%
Central Supply	85–100%
Communications	90–100%
Data Processing	90–100%
Dietary/Food Services	85–100%
Education	85–100%
Fiscal Services	85–100%
Housekeeping	85–100%
Laundry & Linen	85–100%
Maintenance	85–100%
Management Engineering	85–100%
Medical Records	85–100%
Personnel Service	90–100%
Security	90–100%
Social Services	90–100%

Source: From *Productivity and performance management in health care institutions* (1st ed., p. 77) by M. D. McDougal, R. P. Covert, & V. B. Melton, (Eds.), (1989), Chicago: American Hospital Association. Reprinted by permission.

∎ Determine the estimated time spent on indirect (or support) activities per procedure (an example of which is shown in Table 6–6). Multiply the estimated time by Quantity A to compute the total indirect (support) hours (Quantity C).

Table 6–5. Management staffing analysis for an ASLP Department.

Procedure	Volume	×	Labor Standard Hour/Exam	Standard Hours*
Audiological Exam	200	×	1.0	200.0
Hearing Aid Exam	125	×	1.0	125.0
Electronystagmography	75	×	1.5	112.5
Neurodiagnostic(s)	95	×	1.0	95.0
Aural Rehabilitation	60	×	0.5	30.0
Language-Cognitive	90	×	1.0	90.0
Voice-Resonance-Articulation	89	×	1.0	89.0
Dysphagia	75	×	1.0	75.0
Total	809			816.5

Total volume of procedures (A)	A = 809
Total direct hours (B)	B = 816.5
Indirect (support) hours (C) = 0.25 × (A) (at 0.25 hr/procedure in this example)	C = 202.5
Subtotal variable hours required (D) = (B) + (C)	D = 1019
Department utilization target (E) (in this example)	E = 82.1%
Total variable hours required (normalized) (F) = $\frac{(D)}{(E)}$	F = 1241.17
Constant hours (G) (30 days at 24.32 hr/calendar day (in this example)	G = 729.60
Total target worked hours (H) = (F) × (G)	H = 1970.77
Total target FTEs required (I) = (H) divided by 173.33 hr/FTE/month	I = 11.33 FTEs
Vacation/holiday/sick FTE allowance (J) = (I) × 12.5% (percentage varies by hospital department)	J = 1.42 FTEs
Total required paid FTEs (K) = (I) × (J)	K = 12.75 FTEs

* per 30-day period.
Source: Adapted from *Productivity and performance management in health care institutions* (1st ed., p. 78) by M. D. McDougal, R. P. Covert, & V. B. Melton, (Eds.), (1989), Chicago: American Hospital Association.

■ Add Quantity B to Quantity C to determine the subtotal variable hours required (Quantity D).
■ Determine the utilization target (Quantity E) for the ASLP department (as explained in the last section).
■ Divide Quantity D by Quantity E to compute the total variable hours required (Quantity F). This total is "normalized" (i.e., based on a utilization target of 100%) to compare staff requirements of one department with those of other departments in the hospital.
■ Add up the number of staff hours spent per day in fixed activities, such as meetings, classes, inventories, and so forth. Multiply this number by the number of days in the period under

Table 6–6. Quantification of indirect (support) activity in one ASLP Department.

Indirect Activity	Minutes Per Occurrence	Frequency Per Examination	Allocation Time Per Examination (minutes × frequency)
Examination Scheduling	1.5	1.0	1.5
Filing Clerk	2.0	2.0	4.0
Billing	3.0	1.0	3.0
Report Transcription	3.5	1.0	3.5
Hearing Aid follow-up	6.0	.5	3.0
Total support time per examination (in minutes)			15.0

Source: Adapted from *Productivity and performance management in health care institutions* (1st ed., p. 79) by M. D. McDougal, R. P. Covert, & V. B. Melton, (Eds.), (1989), Chicago: American Hospital Association.

study. The result is the total number of hours of fixed activity, or "constant hours" (Quantity G), in the period.

■ Add Quantity F to Quantity G to compute the total target worked hours required (Quantity H).

■ Divide Quantity H by 173.33 (hours per FTE per month in this example) to compute the total target FTEs required (Quantity I).

■ Multiply Quantity I by the percentage of paid staff time in the department for vacation, holiday, and sick leave. The result is the vacation/holiday/sick leave FTE allowance (Quantity J, in FTEs).

■ Add Quantity I to Quantity J (yielding Quantity K) to determine the total required paid FTEs (all positions, flexible (direct), fixed, and, productive). Quantity K is then compared to the actual FTEs paid (including holiday, vacation, and sick days) to determine performance.

When attempting to increase productivity, every alternative should be considered. For example, 40 hr per week (1.0 FTE) can be obtained from a single employee, but can also be achieved through two or more part-time personnel (e.g., 2 × 0.5 FTE = 1.0 FTE). This is particularly useful in situations with less than level workloads, such as higher early morning workload. Utilizing part-time personnel may also allow you to use flex staff (to better accommodate fluctuations in workload) and to allow for hiring of personnel who have previously left the work force (e.g., new mothers) who may not wish full-time employment and whose desired schedule may match workload peaks within the department.

We should look beyond the "FTE is an FTE" mentality and attempt to match activities to skill level. In many instances, departments will be forced to analyze and update the job responsibilities of their current staff and make changes to provide the same (or even better) services at lower cost.

Creativity, and the use of nontraditional ideas, is sometimes difficult to sell in an environment resistant to change. It is ironic that in health care, a field which is undoubtedly experiencing constant change and growth, there may be resistance to changing the fundamental methods by which we accomplish (and even manage) the services we provide. Analyzing the impacts that affect staffing, such as practitioner practice, work flow, and scheduling patterns can be important to developing alternative methods through which we can improve both productivity and the delivery of clinical services.

ASSESSING UTILIZATION OF STAFF AND DEPARTMENTAL PERFORMANCE

Once the utilization target and total required paid FTEs have been determined, ASLP administrators should determine the department's utilization of staff and its performance in comparison with other clinical departments. Utilization of staff is calculated by using the following equation:

$$\text{Utilization of Staff} = \frac{\text{Required Staff (in FTEs)}}{\text{Actual Staff (in FTEs)}}$$

The result of this computation can be incorporated into another equation to determine "normalized performance," a figure that allows managers to compare the performance of one department with that of another. Normalized performance values are based on an organization-wide utilization target of 100%. Normalized performance is computed as follows:

$$\text{Normalized Performance} = \frac{\text{Utilization of Staff}}{\text{Department Utilization Target}}$$

In addition to performing these calculations, ASLP administrators should establish an acceptable operating range using the department utilization target as a midpoint. This range provides the acceptable boundaries of performance for the department and clearly defines performance expectations in advance. An example of computing both utilization of staff and normalized performance for a hypothetical ASLP department is as follows:

> **Required staff = 12.75 FTEs (at 100% utilization)**
> **Actual Staff = 16.00 FTEs**
> **Department utilization target = 82.1%**
> **Acceptable range of performance = Target plus or minus 5%**
>
> $$\text{Utilization of staff} = \frac{12.75}{16.0} = 0.796 = 79.6\%$$

In this example, the utilization of staff was below the utilization target of 82.1% but within the department's acceptable range of performance of 77.1% to 87.1% (or 82.1% plus or minus 5%). Therefore, the utilization of staff within the ASLP department for the period was acceptable.

> $$\text{Normalized performance} = \frac{0.796}{0.821} = 0.969 = 96.9\%$$

In comparison with other hospital departments, the normalized performance was also acceptable. If the normalized operating range of performance determined for this example is 95% (plus or minus 5%), then the value of 96.9% determined here falls within that range.

USING PRODUCTIVITY MONITORING AND REPORTING SYSTEMS

Developing accurate productivity measures is futile without developing an appropriate mechanism to monitor and report department productivity. A productivity monitoring and reporting system is one component of an overall ASLP computer information sytem that can track and evaluate the effectiveness of labor utilization over time. Typical objectives of a productivity monitoring and reporting system include:

∎ Providing department administrators with periodic reports of labor utilization and departmental performance.
∎ Monitoring departmental productivity goals and targets.
∎ Collecting and summarizing the data to be utilized for future planning and budgetary decisions.
∎ Providing timely information that can be used to justify costs, budgets, and reimbursements.
∎ Estimating the impact of new equipment, service delivery, policies and procedures, or regulations on services or budgeted resources.
∎ Providing an indication of those areas where costs can be contained.

A "productivity monitoring and reporting system," then, is a mechanism to report the utilization of staff in a manner that allows management to identify operational fluctuations and make informed decisions. The necessary prerequisites to developing a productivity management report include:

- Actual workload (volume for the period).
- Actual hours worked for the period.
- Actual nonproductive (benefit) hours paid for the period.

Such data form the basis for informal decisions on staff utilization and can enable program administrators to monitor their progress toward greater departmental productivity.

PLANNING FOR CHANGE

Planning for change is important when attempting to optimize resource utilization. Successful change requires a thorough understanding of the operation, its strengths and weaknesses, and an understanding of methodologies to estimate the impact of such change. Another important area to consider is the accurate costing out of the real impact of change. Change is sometimes more far reaching than initially realized. One should never shy away from change, but one must always have a good idea of the associated costs and consequences of that change. Undertaking change without first weighing the associated costs and benefits can be detrimental to the department and to the tenure of the program administrator.

Human nature does not make change easy. Dealing with the "we've always done it that way" attitude is an important barrier to overcome in any improvement project. One should always ask the the following questions: Why is an activity done? Why is it done that way and by those personnel? Answers to questions like these are the single most important function in successfully identifying areas for change. The use of TQM tools can assist in illustrating the inefficiencies inherent in any operation. One aspect of planning which cannot be overemphasized is good communication and feedback with departmental staff. Communication is important for adequately identifying areas for improvement and for anticipating the potential impact of change on the department, specifically, and on the health care organization, in general.

CONCLUSION

Productivity monitoring and operational productivity improvements are not isolated events and should be considered an ongoing and essential component of innovative and progressive management. To maintain the edge, the program administrator must plan for continuous productivity improvement. This facet of managerial responsibility is essential to maintaining the visible, line/staff commitment to change. Productivity and operations improvement activities should be incorporated into an effective departmental action plan. Finally, all department managers and top management should establish appropriate utilization targets and acceptable operating ranges of performance. Setting realistic and achievable goals is important to productivity improvement. In many work environments, formalized employee recognition or reward systems may exist to reward the change desired. Employee reward programs with financial incentives, personal acknowledgements, and quality improvement teams are among the ideas that have been successfully used in the health care industry to encourage desired change. Success stories detailing the actions of innovative organizations are easy to find. However, they all have one thing in common, a desire and willingness to face change and challenge the status quo. Remember, don't rest upon your productivity improvements, build upon them!

REFERENCES

Burack, E. H., & Mathys, N. J. (1979). *Human resources planning: A pragmatic approach to manpower staffing and development.* Lake Forest, IL: Brace-Park Press.

Delbecq, A. L., Van de Ven, A. H., & Gustafson, D. H. (1975). *Group techniques for program planning.* Glenview, IL: Scott Foresman.

Kopelman, R. E. (1986). *Managing productivity in organizations: A practical people-oriented perspective.* New York: McGraw-Hill, Inc.

van Loggerenham, B. J., & Cucchiaro, S. J. (1981). Productivity measurement and the bottom line. *National Productivity Review, 1,* 87–99.

Recommended Readings

Bain, D. (1982). *The productivity prescription.* New York: McGraw-Hill, Inc.

Batten, G. R. (1984). *Enhancing productivity in health care facilities.* Owings Mills, MD: National Health Publishing.

Gray, S. P., & Steffy, W. (1983). *Hospital cost containment through productivity management.* New York: Van Nostrand Reinhold Co.

Hanks, K. (1986). *Up your productivity.* Los Altos, CA: William Kaufmann, Inc.

Kirk, R. (1988). *Healthcare quality & productivity: Practical management tools.* Rockville, MD: Aspen Publishers, Inc.

McConnell, C. R. (1986). *The health care supervisor's guide to cost control and productivity improvement.* Rockville, MD: Aspen Systems Corp.

McDougal, M. D., Covert, R. P., & Melton,V. B. (Eds.). (1989). *Productivity and performance management in health care institutions.* Chicago, IL: American Hospital Publishing, Inc.

Riggs, J. L., & Felix, G. H. (1983). *Productivity by objectives: Results-oriented solutions to the productivity puzzle.* Englewood Cliffs, NJ: Prentice-Hall Inc.

Simon, S. E. (1983). Work measurement methods: An approach to productivity management in human services. *Journal of Rehabilitation Administration, 7,* 151–163.

Smalley, H. E. (1982). *Hospital management engineering: A guide to the improvement of hospital management systems.* Englewood Cliffs, NJ: Prentice-Hall Inc.

Templin, J. L. (1983). Productivity in the supervisor. *Health Care Supervisor, 1,* 1–11.

Source Of Additional Information

The Healthcare Information and Management Systems Society (HIMSS) of the American Hospital Association has numerous publications and papers related to health care systems, productivity improvement, and operations analysis. Further information can be obtained by contacting the HIMSS, 840 North Lake Shore Drive, Chicago, IL 60611, (312) 280-6148.

7

COMPUTERIZED INFORMATION SYSTEMS

Kenneth W. Heard, PhD

"*The real danger of our technological age is not so much that machines will begin to think like men, but that men begin to think like machines.*"

(Sydney J. Harris, Publishers Newspaper Syndicate)

With the arrival of computer technology for administrative applications, department managers have achieved new levels in program automation (e.g., for viewing patient demographic data, treatment, billing, and managing productivity). Computer usage in ASLP has changed significantly (Shewan, 1989) due to considerable improvements in personal computers (PCs), reduced cost, and the availability of software packages for clinical application. PCs appear in ASLP programs through equipment manufacturers who have developed computer-based diagnostic and therapeutic treatment protocols.

Computerized information systems (ISs) are becoming increasingly important because health care organizations are turning their focus from departmental to organizational automation and from financial to patient-care applications (Lafferty, 1987). Today, most ISs are part of a predetermined plan that integrates clinical, administrative, and financial data with a communications network that combines these three components (Fournier & Margolis, 1991).

Administrators need to know that the IS in, or to be installed in, the department can meet program specifications. If it cannot, it is probably because the components to do so are not contained in the computer system that was purchased. The risk and cost in choosing the wrong IS are rising dramatically. Administrative and patient-care applications require major investments in equipment, computer systems personnel, staff, and user training. If the department discovers after the initial installation that it is unable to integrate the IS totally, it can become a major financial issue to correct.

This chapter will present some of the salient issues that face program administrators and their staff concerning computerized ISs. The author will provide the reader with insight into the value of computers in ASLP settings, to help define departmental needs, and devise a practical approach to integrate such systems to fulfill program objectives.

DESIGNING A SYSTEM

Successful integration of ISs demands advanced planning (Meyer & Sunquist, 1986). An IS should be chosen only after a department has completely surveyed its needs and priorities. This process will identify the size of the IS, power requirements, and the amount of information sharing that must be available both in/outside of the department. The planning process should involve representatives from ASLP, the computer information department (if available), or a computer consultant (see Appendix 7A, "Choosing a consultant") to address IS needs and to stimulate thinking of the staff concerning computers. For example, staff members should be asked the following questions:

- Briefly describe your responsibilities within the department.
- Briefly describe how computers assist you in meeting responsibilities. What is your level of computer literacy?
- What are the major advantages to using computers?
- What is your primary source of information concerning computers (e.g., professional association, user groups, magazines, self-teaching, etc.)?
- What reporting mechanism do you need to enhance job performance?
- How do you keep track of information (e.g., manual or automated systems)?
- What major concerns do you have in the use of computers?
- What actions should be taken to overcome these concerns?

- What are your short-and-long range expectations of computer systems?
- What should the hardware/software be expected to do for you?

The survey will prevent the committee from making nearsighted judgments concerning size, purpose, and future expansion. Several other considerations that the survey should address are:

- Data transmission with insurance companies and other financial affiliations (e.g., credit agencies, banks, investments);
- Access to distributors of office supplies, clinical equipment, electronic messages, patient-care data base programs;
- Clinical applications for patient assessment/treatment and for patient education;
- Office automation (word processing, spreadsheets, graphics, and database management).

This approach will identify all software requirements first (Hoffman, 1985). Based on these findings, the IS study team should develop a series of recommendations to solve technical and nontechnical problems. From these requirements, the ASLP administrator will develop a request for proposal (RFP) that defines the IS to be installed by the vendor. The RFP is sent to vendors who have ISs that meet the department's expectations. Then the program administrator will review and select bids that merit further evaluation. Finally, a format should be developed for presenting the benefits of the plan to top management (if applicable). The interest and support of both administration and users of the IS are essential to its success. Utilizing professionals from university-based affiliations can provide a good opportunity to draw upon resources of the academic community and to strengthen collaborative relationships between educators and health care providers.

Years ago, ISs were based upon designs shown in Figure 7–1. This illustration displays what was typically found in large organizations where there was a high degree of departmental/interdepartmental information sharing. Departmental needs were usually restricted to stand-alone PCs, with no information sharing (*lower left*), and steadily progressed to limited, general, and total information sharing largely attributed to maxi-and-miniframe installations (*upper right*, respectively). However, total information sharing can now be achieved through the computing power of individual PCs which can be connected to other systems. ISs can be categorized as follows:

- Independent systems use stand-alone software programs to access information of interest to the originating department. Although these programs can be modified, communication between workstations is prohibited.
- Centralized systems allow information to be transmitted between departments simultaneously, using software packages that

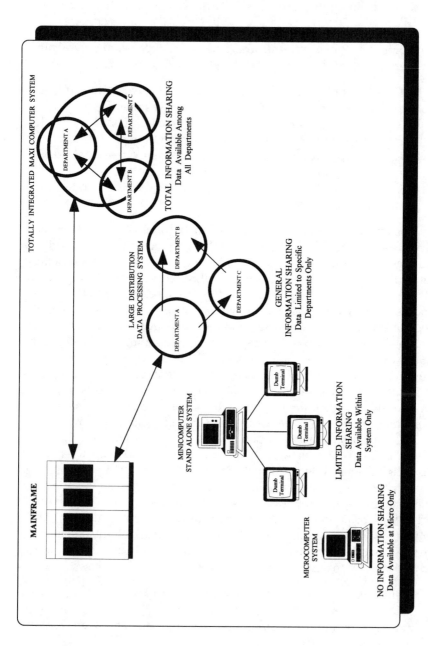

Figure 7–1. Graphic representation of the levels of computing power and data sharing.

ensure data accessibility, security, and integrity. However, a department's dependence upon centralized databases is limited.
∎ Distributed systems are customized departmental systems that can be shared with other departments. This system is most suitable in ASLP because it is independent of organizational mainframes and data sharing can be controlled by the originating department.

Sharrott (1991) reports that central and distributed systems are usually installed in corporate organizations.

Should ASLP programs be fortunate enough to develop an IS from inception, many hardware/software compatibility issues can be avoided. Unfortunately, many ISs are patched together over time, using different computer components. Hence, predetermined knowledge of the different levels of computing power available, and the degree of connectivity (i.e., the extent to which a given computer or program can function in a network setting), is a prerequisite.

SOFTWARE SELECTION

There are two software alternatives once the decision has been made to purchase a computer system, regardless of its application. The first alternative is to develop the software in house. Although this process usually does not require large software expenditures from the department's budget, it may require considerable expenditure from the operating budget of the computer systems department for the time required of these specialists involved in design and development. For ASLP organizations without a computer systems department, this likely involves outside contracting for systems design services. Although in house development involves considerable start-up time, the end product is generally unique to the needs of that particular program, as well as to its philosophy, and practices. Furthermore, the decision regarding the level of integration of the software with existing ISs remains within the organization.

The second alternative is to purchase a software package from a commercial vendor. These packages fall into two categories. General-purpose software (e.g., EXCEL, dBASE) provides the user with a framework that can be revised to meet future requirements and expectations. Special-purpose software, on the other hand, is designed for a particular application or group of applications. In most cases, purchased software packages are designed for stand-alone PCs. These systems are usually packaged to provide a variety of support during the implementation phase. The support offered by the vendor usually consists of user training and, in some instances, software program modifications to customize the applications to the unique requirements of the clinic. Some vendors, for an additional cost, extend these services to accommodate future expectations. However, caution should be exercised in these agreements. Prospective buyers may be lured into purchasing a service contract based on promises for future technology and innovation that may never materialize. The IS should be evaluated based on its existing potential, not on what it may or may not be capable of doing in the future.

Decisions must be made concerning the development (if applicable), purchase, installation, and staff training in the use of various types of software modules: financial management, human resource management, materiels management, quality improvement, office automation, and multiuser automation, and so forth.

Financial Management

Financial management programs are software systems (usually more than one program) that can be used to keep all of a business's financial records on a PC. They usually are built around a general ledger program, and include options for printing bills, checks, profit/loss statements, and balance sheets. Many large customized accounting packages are available. As with almost all accounting packages, the user must know general bookkeeping principles to use this program.

Financial management programs (e.g., PeachTree Complete III, PeachTree Software, Inc.) often consist of various modules that can be designed to meet the specific needs of the ASLP practice. These programs can create and maintain files of financial transactions including additions to and subtractions from specific reimbursement accounts. Furthermore, the financial management functions of a general ledger system can allow the comparison of income/expenses as well as the generation of reports by clinical specialty. Most general accounting ledgers allow the user to develop comparative year-to-date reports, along with proposed budgets or cash flow reports. Financial management software can allow the user to generate customized financial reports or modify reports to meet the specific needs of the practice. These programs provide maximum flexibility in developing financial statements without any significant expense for customizing an income statement.

Patient billing programs are designed to generate itemized patient billing statements, prepare patient bills for insurance filing, generate automatic aging reports which list all delinquent/open accounts, and account history reports. For further discussion of financial management, see Chapter 8.

Human Resource Management (HRM)

HRM software maintains personnel data to assist management in forecasting and long-range planning efforts. These systems are designed to: (1) perform pay-rate calculations; (2) determine eligibility for fringe benefits; (3) distribute costs to individual accounts; (4) generate labor and cost analysis reports by specialty function; and (5) generate statistics on employee turnover, absenteeism, use of overtime, and productivity.

Staffing the ASLP department probably represents a major portion of the program's operating costs, accounting for 40% or more of the entire clinic's budget. ISs can play a key role in providing accurate, relevant information for use in administrative decision making related to the largest components of the clinic budget. These software programs will flag information that falls outside (above or below) a specified range. This feature avoids burdening the ASLP administrator with voluminous reports and redirects attention to potential problems. If maintained, these personal data bases can supply information to fulfill a variety of functions. Administrators will have current access to records for performance appraisal purposes and are readily accessible to monitor clinical compliance for accreditation purposes. For an in-depth discussion on human resource management, the reader is referred to Chapter 4.

Staff utilization and scheduling are another administrative area to which computer technology has been applied. The objective of these systems is to monitor services and to ensure that they are available when needed. These packages can be designed to assist in scheduling test rooms by clinicians, and in making advanced appointments. Each department specialty and clinician defines the parameters that are unique to that area. The software then generates a listing of the availability of that specialty or provider for appointments, open schedules status reports, patient reminders, and statistics regarding staff utilization, as well as other reports that can assist managers in the efficient allocation of clinic resources.

Materiel Management

Materiel inventory and purchasing programs are designed to maintain a perpetual inventory by unit item, supplier, dollar amount, and estimate the anticipated amount of time over which the inventory item will be depleted. These packages are also capable of automatically generating purchasing orders as unit items are depleted and they can provide an analysis of usage and unit cost.

Quality Improvement

The process of establishing and monitoring the quality of care provided has become a key issue in the delivery of ASLP health care. Increasingly sophisticated quality improvement programs have been implemented in organizations in response to increased consumer awareness regarding ASLP, more stringent accreditation guidelines, rising costs of health care, and pressure from peer review to support the growing professionalism of ASLP. For further discussion on quality improvement (QI), refer to Chapter 5.

While the author is unaware of any software programs to measure quality of care, ASLP administrators might experience difficulty substantiating the validity of such a tool within their own organizations. The aspects of care prescribed by a vendor might be inconsistent with those established by the ASLP organization regarding the appropriateness of the indicators used to evaluate those standards. Therefore, many ASLP administrators should continue to carry on with their existing monitoring practices while taking advantage of ISs to process and summarize the data collected (Schifiliti, Bonasero, & Thompson, 1986). However, the real opportunities for automated quality improvement applications exist with networked ISs (to be discussed in the next section). Relying on computerized ASLP plans and patient care documentation, using networked systems, administrators have the capability to retrieve on-line data rapidly, which saves considerable time.

Office Automation

Office automation is the application of computer and communications technology to office activities. It is by no means restricted to administrative offices. It has the potential to affect almost every aspect of office work, including text processing, filing, telephone communications, personal planning, messaging, and meetings. The major office automation systems currently utilized are word processing and electronic mail (E-mail), database management programs, electronic spreadsheet programs, and graphics programs. Software programs that combine two or more of these software functions are referred to as an integrated software program.

Many computer users ask, "What is the best word processing software?" The answer depends upon compatibility issues, department networking plans, and departmental users who are familiar with its application. Having experienced users of a particular package will expedite in house training of all staff members which will achieve effective utilization of that software program. (This criterion can also apply to the selection of other software packages.) If in house experts are unavailable, the administrator must consider the costs of hiring a consultant to train the staff to facilitate the learning process.

Multiuser Automation

Network hardware and operating systems provide the capability of connecting different types of computers to the same network, and different local or remote networks to each other. Networks must be supported by specific software requirements which are called network operating systems (NOS). When properly installed, users can access and share data with other users. This approach is possible but not without considerable headaches and greater cost for installation and management. If MS DOS-based systems and MacIntosh-based systems are used on the same network, additional software requirements must be met so that the information obtained or generated by one system is accessible and readable by the another system.

NETWORKING

Local area network (LAN) describes a routine for using PCs to communicate with each other in the absence of hardware/software related problems. The goal of networking is to allow users to exchange information, share peripherals (e.g., laser printers), and draw on the resources of a large secondary storage unit (file server). LANs provide the advantage of a distributed IS in which computer power is distributed to users without compromising their ability to communicate via electronic mail to share multiuser programs and to access shared databases.

Some of the largest and most complex LANS are housed in university and health care organizations. These networks may be comprised of several smaller networks connected by electronic bridges (devices that allow two networks to exchange data). Unlike a multiuser system, in which each user is provided with a dumb terminal that may lack processing capabilities, each user in a LAN has a workstation containing its own processing circuitry. High-speed communication cables connect these workstations. Designated network protocols (e.g., AppleTalk and EtherNet) control the flow of information within the networks. These protocols determine when and how a node (connection point in a LAN that creates, receives, or repeats a message) may initiate a message. Network protocols can manage conflicts that occur when two nodes transmit information at the same time.

The basic elements of a LAN are cables, a network interface card (an adapter that couples a network cable to a PC), a file server (a PC that provides access to files for all workstations in the network), a network operating system (system software that links the networks hardware components), and PCs or workstations linked by the system. Network topology refers to the geometric arrangement of computers in a LAN. Common topologies for interconnecting workstations include:

- ■ Bus network. Cables run from computer to computer simultaneously. Each node in the network, however, has a unique address and receiver circuitry which monitors the bus to determine whether a message is being sent to the node (e.g., a message sent to a printer node is overlooked by the other nodes in the network).
- ■ Ring network. Nodes (e.g., workstations, peripherals, and file servers) are arranged around a closed loop cable.
- ■ Star network. A centralized network with the physical layout of a star. Nodes are connected directly to the central processor located in the center.

Deciding upon the proper type of network topology depends upon current and future functional needs. The most frustrating experience is to purchase a computer network system and then find out that the system is incapable of handling additional users without tremendous costs, or that it cannot provide additional network functions deemed essential after the system is operational.

The everyday user who graduates from a stand-alone computer system to multiuser system should hardly notice that he or she has become part of a network except, of course, for the benefit of better access to data exchange. The role of database administration, however, becomes naturally more delicate and important in the network environment, as optimal performance, data security, and the integrity of data are essential for long-term use of the network. For this reason, a well-planned system of control within the database system must be introduced. This will make it possible to clearly define and control who has access to what data and what each user can do at the administrative, clinical, and office operations level. In this way, software-related conflicts among users within the network can be prevented regardless of whether the department is using a high-end (expensive) or low-end (inexpensive) network operating system. State-of-the-art LANs provide communication (connectivity) to promote data sharing with other staff members.

MS-DOS systems can communicate with Macintosh systems via a gateway (a device that connects two dissimilar LANs through a protocol conversion) as shown in Figure 7–2. This hardware configuration, however, has some drawbacks such as increased costs of LAN installation, reduced effectiveness of some workstations due to "RAM CRAM" (i.e., additional device drivers are required to support communication), and much slower performance from emulation software (duplicates the functional capability of one device in another device). Although IBM compatible software can run on Macintosh computers using emulation software (e.g., SoftPC), the program's execution speed will be greatly reduced. Given the tremendous speed of 386 and 486-based microcomputers, users who are accustomed to such speed for data, graphics, and text-based applications may be adversely affected by the much slower performance in the emulation mode. Departments that have different computers in use must decide if networking these systems is cost effective.

Any department that plans to network with other programs must ensure its capacity to expand and communicate within the organization. This requires an understanding of the hardware platform in use throughout the system. A hardware platform is a computer standard, such as IBM-PC compatible or Macintosh PC, in which an in-depth approach to solving computer problems is based. Standards (ANSI) have been developed to provide greater networking opportunities for different computer systems to access information on similar or different networks (Derfler, 1991; Derfler, 1992; Dunbar, 1990). This design allows various dedicated networks to be linked to a centralized system or to other organization-wide networks (Figure 7–3).

The demand for connectivity between different systems, networks, and hardware platforms has made this area of development a rapidly growing

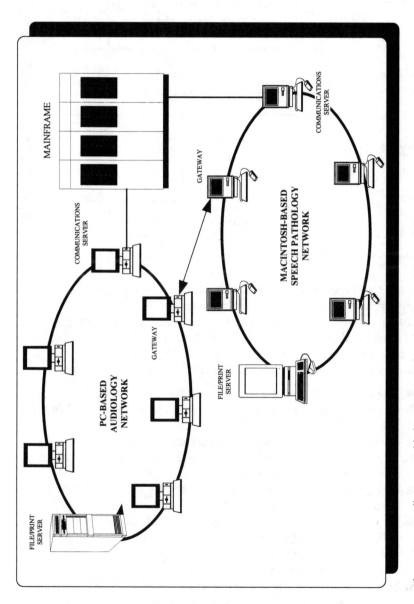

Figure 7–2. An illustration of linking MS-DOS based systems to Macintosh-based systems with access to host systems (mainframes).

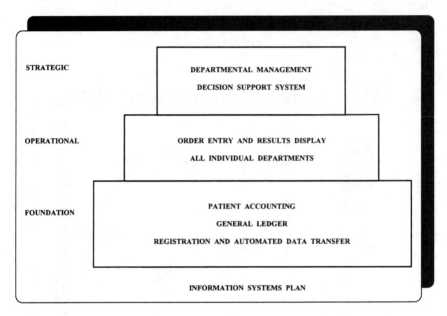

STRATEGIC

DEPARTMENTAL MANAGEMENT

DECISION SUPPORT SYSTEM

OPERATIONAL

ORDER ENTRY AND RESULTS DISPLAY

ALL INDIVIDUAL DEPARTMENTS

FOUNDATION

PATIENT ACCOUNTING

GENERAL LEDGER

REGISTRATION AND AUTOMATED DATA TRANSFER

INFORMATION SYSTEMS PLAN

Figure 7–3. An example of the hierarchy of information systems within a health care organization.

market in the computer industry. Departments can computerize their operations in the absence of constraints imposed by large organizations. The department's survey may require that a high-end LAN operating system (e.g., Novell's Netware, Microsoft LAN Manager, IBM LAN Server, and Banyan Systems Inc.'s Vines, etc.) be installed. The following factors dictate whether a department will need a high-end LAN operating software:

- The number of workstations is more than 50.
- The department needs to connect to remote devices and organizational ISs.
- Users need to access the LAN from remote locations.
- The system requires local or remote LANs (LAN-to-LAN) to be linked together via electronic bridges.
- Macintosh-based systems need to be integrated with MS DOS-based systems in the same LAN.
- Host mainframe connections are required for the users on the ASLP LAN. (In a computer network, the computer that performs centralized functions such as making programs or data files available to workstations in the network.)
- System fault tolerance is required on the ASLP LAN to ensure data integrity (i.e., when the system goes down it has some tolerance to return back to its active state).
- A dozen, or more, users require access to the same files.

- ■ Shared security access rights are assigned to individual users as defined by the network administrator.
- ■ Audit trail services that monitor file servers and the actions they require are needed.

While ASLP equipment manufacturers provide "turnkey" software applications for the private practitioner, their use has been primarily for stand-alone operations and are not LAN compatible. For many years, manufacturers have provided computer interface capabilities to clinical equipment. However, without network compatibility, the buyer could be spending an additional $2,000–$3,000 for a system that displays and stores equipment-specific data only. Furthermore, most clinical software requires ASLPs to enter patient data manually for each diagnostic system used. This is contrary to the primary purpose of an integrated IS which is to enter data only once. Given the benefits of LANs, it seems ludicrous to purchase computer-based ASLP equipment that is not network compatible. Vendors are, however, reportedly addressing this issue.

LANs can fulfill professional and current legislative requirements such as: (1) the management of quality clinical services, which is becoming a generally recognized obligation; (2) the consolidation of documents and data for clinics regarding patients, treatment procedures, and the duration of treatment which are required as a basis for reimbursement with third-party payers; and (3) the improvement of efficiency in clinical operations (Koyanagi, Nakahara, Hirose, Hori, & Nakano, 1989; Friedman & Dieterle, 1990; Hekelman, Kelly, & Grundner, 1990).

COMPUTERIZED AUDIOLOGY DEPARTMENTS

The author wishes to report the results of a computerized audiology network in use (Figure 7–4), since 1986, at the John L. McClellan Veterans Hospital, Little Rock, Arkansas. The IS was first established as an audiological network which linked five diagnostic audiometers (located in Little Rock) to PCs for collecting and storing patient data on a central file server, and for generating patient reports. Since then, another LAN has been installed in another clinical division located in North Little Rock. Both divisions communicate with each other through a remote bridge (a device that allows two networks to exchange data) via the hospital microwave system. For example, ASLP patients are seen at one division for diagnostic evaluations with follow-up rehabilitation being completed at the second division. Patients have been known to appear at one site while their clinical records are housed at the other facility. The network system allows the staff to retrieve relevant test results, progress notes,

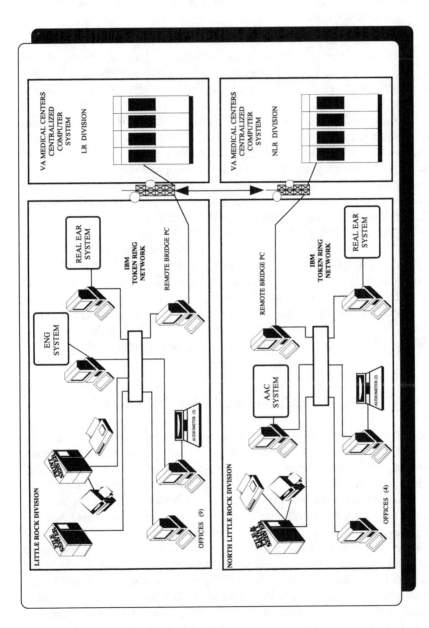

Figure 7-4. An illustration of the John L. McClellan VA Medical Center Audiology Service PC network.

and reports that are stored on the other division's file server. Since the ASLP staff has joint appointments at both divisions, the remote bridge permits easy access to patient data regardless of the work site. The network also provides access to specialized application software (e.g., word processing, dBASE, spreadsheets, and graphics). We can access clinical data immediately, thereby eliminating the difficulties inherent in data acquisition from the hospital's centralized system. Minimal programming time was required to design a patient database management system (PDMS) and computer interface to the audiology equipment.

Administrative management has been enhanced through a patient tracking system which records provider workloads taken from patient charge slips that are related to CPT code terminology. A compiled inventory of all patient visits, patient demographics, case mix statistics, clinician productivity, hearing aid stock, and progress note entries are available through the network's database. These tabulations can be obtained in a few minutes. Previously, data analysis took three individuals approximately two days per month to complete. Thus, the same work can be done and the same output is guaranteed, but it is carried out in a different and more efficient way. A LAN allows file servers, printers, and other devices to be shared, which represents another aspect of cost containment.

Several publications (Fournier & Margolis, 1991; Margolis & Thornton, 1991) have reported the benefits to be derived from networking clinical environments. The selection of diagnostic and therapeutic software should consider the networking hardware/software compatibility issues previously discussed. These experiences should provide insight into the development of standard protocols for networking ASLP environments.

IMPROVING PRODUCTIVITY THROUGH INFORMATION SYSTEMS

Today, ASLPs work in a competitive, cost-constrained environment where issues related to quality and productivity have become a matter of financial and organizational survival. ISs can be used to monitor staff productivity, program management, cost containment, and quality of care. For example, the department manager might review weekly statistics on patient visits for specific procedures, patient billing data, and clinic cost data. Graphics software could be used to display patterns in the data (e.g., projections of patient appointment times/day and utilization under assumptions based on present trends). These findings can reveal the effect of a number of important variables (e.g., age of the population served, procedures performed, and market share). Assumptions concerning market share would then be adjusted to account for utilization rate to changes in the market share (to be discussed in Chapter 9). Several examples of ISs that monitor staff productivity have been developed for MS DOS and Macintosh-based systems (Margolis & Thornton, 1991). For an in-depth discussion on managing productivity, the reader is referred to Chapter 6.

SECURITY AND CONFIDENTIALITY

The use of ISs increases the complexity of maintaining patient confidentiality. IS security comprises both physical (or nonphysical) and intentional (or nonintentional) threats to systems integrity. Universal concerns about patient confidentiality constitute a commonly accepted standard of ethical practice. A breech of IS confidentiality refers to the disclosure of information stored in a computer to an unauthorized source. If computer networks are to be beneficial to the delivery of ASLP services, everyone from the department manager on down must be sensitized to this matter. The National Independent Study Center (1992) reports a variety of methods to maintain confidentiality of computer-stored data.

While computerized records appear vulnerable to breaches in security, a properly designed IS (or LAN) can restrict unauthorized access. For example, if someone violates a system's security code and gains illegal access, a security module can automatically track and record this activity. The security module operates whenever the computer system is powered. This is unlike hand-written medical records which have limited surveillance once they are removed from the filing system.

Low-end LAN software can provide workstation-specific access only (as opposed to user-specific access). Workstation-specific access refers to logging onto the network at an authorized site to view a specific database on the file server. For example, a user could access financial records, but only from the computer housed in the office of the manager. The primary disadvantage of workstation-specific access is that security is reduced when a particular site is powered (i.e., any user can access information available at that workstation).

High-end LAN software provides individual users with varying levels of access. Here, departmental users log onto the system through private access codes. A network administrator (the person responsible for maintaining the network and assisting end users) defines the application and database access for each user regardless of where the person logs onto the system. Once the users log on, they can access their assigned data despite the location of the terminal.

During the system design phase (previously discussed), the IS study group must consider the level of employee access to select databases and the type of security system to be installed. High-end security systems can control access to patient records (this may not be the case with low-end systems). Presently, client-server (searching for a specific database) management software programs for LANs provide greater security of information that cannot be circumvented even at the LAN's file server station (a computer that provides services for users of the network). All requests for data stored on the file server must past through the server software, eliminating the need for keyboard commands to bypass security (Buzzard, 1990).

ASLP departments communicate considerable information to regulate the appropriate usage of IS. Each employee must understand the department's overall policy, and that of its medical center (if appropriate), preferred procedures, levels of responsibility and accountability, communication, and potential problems. A security policy should be prepared and maintained in the ASLP policy and procedure manual (see Appendixes 7B and 7C).

Securing a particular database must include site, backup, and recovery procedures. The computer environment must be protected from the occurrence of natural disasters (e.g., fire, storms, flooding, etc.). Furthermore, the central processing area should be secured from unauthorized access by outsiders. This may require a secured (locked) computer room, PC, or file server when the area is unattended. Less efficient security methods consist of special booting programs (e.g., PC Disklock) located at each workstation.

Scheduled backup procedures are absolutely necessary when using ISs (Mendelson, 1989). All users must establish a backup of their applications, data, and private information. The time required to restore a system is minimal compared to the time required to reenter data into the computer. The frequency of backup depends on the amount of information entered or revised and level of importance. Daily backups of the clinic file server or central mass storage are highly recommended. The backup copy should be stored off-site to prevent a disaster to the original and backup copies. A general rule of thumb is if the data expand beyond 40 megabytes (MB) of storage, the user should consider using a tape backup system instead of high-capacity floppy diskettes (Mendelson). Backup system software packages can be directed to tape or optical disk drives to prevent taking a workstation or file server off-line during a backup procedure. Backups which take more than 30 minutes (for large file servers) should be scheduled during evening or lunch hours.

A LOOK INTO THE FUTURE

Today's technology has improved the performance of desktop computers to approximate performance consistent with mini-and-mainframe systems. Advances in technology appear in semi-annual, quarterly, and even monthly periodicals. These advances have been in CPU processing, disk storage capacity, reduced costs, integrated software programs, communications, networking, and so forth.

Health care organizations are moving to PC-based network file servers and workstations to customize ISs installed in clinical departments. Contingent upon adequate funding, these departments can be structured to interface clinical and computer-based systems into a LAN. More complex LANs could be connected to special workgroups (e.g., LAN audiology test suites, LAN SLP treatment rooms, LAN research labs, LAN business management offices, etc.). Here, LANs could access one another (horizontally) via gateways while the department IS communicates vertically with hospital or university mainframe systems. The technology to install this architecture is available. Manufacturers who provide hardware/software related products to the ASLP profession must continue to keep pace with this rapidly changing industry. They must design systems to function in a networked environment instead of costly stand-alone systems that lack network capabilities.

SUMMARY

ISs presage a new era in health care practice. A systematic process for the introduction of ISs into clinical departments has been described. The enlightened use of ISs in clinics may help us achieve a new state-of-the-art in ASLP. Administrators and their staff should be sensitive to the potential impact of ISs on job satisfaction. While a complete IS may not be for every clinical environment, under the right circumstances, such a system can be a joy to use. The essential ingredients include the right personalities, a supportive staff, a good vendor, and superior hardware/software to make it work. The author is of the opinion that the potential is truly worth the quest.

REFERENCES

Buzzard, J. (1990). *Database server evaluation guide:* An independent survey. San Francisco, CA: Hammerhead System.

Derfler, F. J., Jr. (1991). *Guide to connectivity.* Berkley, CA: ZD Press.

Derfler, F. J., Jr. (1992). Connectivity simplified. *PC Magazine,* March, 251–293.

Dunbar, C. (1990). The networking standards evolution: Toward a real electronic medical record. *Computers in Healthcare, 11,* 18–21.

Fournier, E., & Margolis, R. (1991). A microcomputer networked audiology clinic. *Audiology Today, 3,* 28–31.

Friedman, B. A., & Dieterle, R. C. (1990). Integrating information systems in hospitals. *Archives of Pathology and Laboratory Medicine, 114,* 13–15.

Ginsberg, M. (1992). Finding and keeping a quality computer consultant. *Audiology Today, 4,* 35–37.

Hekelman, F. P., Kelly, R., & Grundner, T. M. (1990). Computerized health information networks: House calls of the future. *Family Medicine, 22,* 392–395.

Hoffman, F. M. (1985). Evaluating and selecting a computer software package. *Journal of Nursing Education, 18,* 51–55.

Koyanagi, T., Nakahara, H., Hirose, K., Hori, E., & Nakano, H. (1989). A 2-year assessment of a microcomputer based local-area network system for managing perinatal medical information. *International Journal of Bio-Medical Computing, 24,* 257–268.

Lafferty, K. D. (1987). Patient care systems versus financial systems: The cost justification battle. *Nursing Management, 18*, 51–56.

Margolis, R., & Thornton, A. R. (1991). Spreadsheet systems for tracking audiology patients. *Audiology Today, 3*, 24–26.

Mendelson, E. (1989). Backup software. *PC Magazine, 14*, 269–272.

Meyer, D., & Sunquist, J. (1986). Selecting a management system. *Computers in Healthcare, 7*, 22–24.

National Independent Study Center. (1992). Computer Security Awareness training materials: Independent study package. Denver, CO: U.S. Office of Personnel Management.

Palmer, C. (1990). Computer applications in audiology. *Audiology Today, 2*, 27–28.

Schifiliti, C., Bonasero, C., & Thompson, M. (1986). Lotus 1-2-3: A quality assurance application for nursing practice, administration, and staff development. *Computers in Nursing, 4*, 205–211.

Sharrott, L. A. (1991). Centralized and distributed information systems: Two Architecture Approaches for the 90s. In M.J. Ball, J.V. Douglas, R. I. O'Desky, & J. W. Albright (Eds), *Healthcare information management systems.* New York: Springer-Verlag.

Shewan, C. M. (1989). Computer usage on the rise. *Asha, 31*, 35.

Recommended Readings

Childs, B. W. (1991). Consulting: State of the art. In M. J. Ball, J. V. Douglas, R. I. O'Desky, & J. W. Albright (Eds), *Healthcare information management systems.* New York: Springer-Verlag.

Convey, H. D., Craven, N. H., & McAlister, N. H., (1985). *Concepts and issues in health care computing.* St. Louis, MO: C.V. Mosby Company.

Gans, D.N. (1989). Medical group information system. *Journal of the Medical Group Management Association, 11*, 55–56.

Mikuleky, M. P., & Ledford, C. (1987). *Computers in nursing, hospital, and clinical applications.* Reading, MA: Addison-Wesley Publishing Company, Inc.

Schmitz, H. H. (1979). *Hospital information systems.* Germantown, MD: Aspen Systems Corporation.

APPENDIX 7A

Choosing a Consultant

Ginsberg (1992) describes three types of IS consultants that can be enlisted for different purposes:

- **General consultants** handle general hardware, software, and purchasing problems for the department.
- **Training consultants** provide onsite demonstrations to the staff on specific types of software programs. The benefits to be realized here will improve the staff's learning curve when introducing new equipment and procedures.
- **Programming consultants** can provide customized software for ASLP applications. Although commercially available, software packages for ASLP practice may require customizing to be configured for specific applications.

Selecting the right consultant can be a difficult challenge for an administrator. A thorough interview should disclose previous work experiences (with references), work ethic, and level of education. This will establish the consultant's track record, level of enthusiasm, and any biases toward personal selection of computer hardware, software, or vendors. (Objectivity may be difficult to maintain if the consultant represents a particular vendor.) The administrator needs to determine if the consultant is experienced in mini/mainframe systems design to develop a PC-based network system. Should the consultant represent a large firm, knowledge of who will be providing the service must be determined.

Palmer (1990) gives us a list of helpful questions applicable to prospective consultant(s):

- What is the exact cost (or best estimate) for services?
- Will customized software be designed for the clinic (i.e., patient database or record control)?
- Will educational training be provided to the staff in the use of the hardware/software? Is there an extra fee for training? Will user friendly documentation be provided?
- How will the IS be purchased (i.e., through competitive pricing or based on the consultant's recommendations)?
- Will the consultant install the equipment?
- Will the consultant be available to support future hardware or software concerns? What is the response turnaround time? What is the cost?

- Will periodic newsletters be available to update the users about the computer system?
- Can the consultant provide a list of sources who have used his/her service(s)?

APPENDIX 7B

Information System (IS) Security—Sample

The following information system security policy is adapted from the Audiology and Speech Pathology Service, Department of Veterans Affairs, Chillicothe, Ohio, submitted by Stephen R. Rizzo, Jr., PhD.

1. PURPOSE: To establish ASLP Service policy, procedure and responsibility in IS Security.
2. POLICY: It is the policy of ASLP Service that computer hardware and software will be protected from unauthorized access, loss, or destruction; that data integrity, system reliability, and data availability will be maintained, and that data disclosure will be released only by authorized individuals.
3. RESPONSIBILITIES:
   a. The ASLP administrator is responsible for the implementation of the principles and policies contained in the Medical Center's IS Security Memorandum and may delegate appropriate responsibilities to supervisors and/or the department computer systems coordinator.
   b. The ASLP administrator is responsible for:
      (1) recommending assignments of new access to systems and level of access required.
      (2) training of end users in the proper use of IS equipment and the related IS security policies and procedures.
      (3) supervising the use of IS equipment.
      (4) providing data validation and protection of data from loss or unauthorized release
      (5) identifying and reporting actual or suspected security breaches to the Medical Center's IS Security Officer.
      (6) ensuring that the computer systems and personnel departments are properly informed when the employment status of an IS user of this department changes.
   c. Staff members are responsible for adhering to established medical center and department policies and procedures in regards to networked IS security.
4. PROCEDURES:
   a. Identification of all ISs and responsible staff. For ease in updating, this information is provided in Appendix 7C.
   b. System Access:
      (1) For the ASLP system, the program administrator will initiate requests for system access utilizing the principle of least privileges.

(2) Each employee of this service who has access to an IS that requires the use of authorization codes is responsible for safeguarding those codes. Security codes will be memorized (will not be written or recorded) and will never be divulged to any other person except as identified in the signed IS Security Access Agreement.

(3) The ASLP administrator will ensure that proper action is taken when there is change in the user's employment status. All notifications will be accomplished within one work day of the employment action.

c. Personnel Security Management:

(1) The ASLP administrator will perform a careful job analysis for all positions to determine the position sensitivity level.

(2) The ASLP administrator will review for each job, utilizing the principle of least privileges and the menu options needed for carrying out the required jobs, and will recommend the appropriate level of access.

(3) The ASLP administrator will ensure that position descriptions and performance standards of each position requiring access to sensitive data reflect appropriate statements regarding IS security.

(4) The ASLP administrator will annually review the position description and performance standards regarding IS security and the consequences of noncompliance will be addressed in the review.

d. IS Security Awareness:

(1) The ASLP administrator will develop and implement a security awareness training program that addresses, at a minimum, the definition of information security relationship of IS security procedures to the employee's specific responsibilities, consequences for inadvertent or intentional security breach, the IS security policy of the medical center and ASLP Service, purpose of information security, how to report security concerns, and procedures for logging off systems (this could be addressed and appropriately documented in service staff meetings).

(2) The ASLP administrator will ensure that each employee who has access to networked IS sensitive information receives continuing IS security training as it relates to the requirements of the employee's duties. At a minimum, annual training is required (this could be addressed and appropriately documented in service staff meetings).

(3) The ASLP administrator will ensure that IS security awareness training is provided at the time of initial employment/

assignment and before the issuance of authorization codes and that the employee has had the opportunity to read the medical center's IS security policy and guidelines (if applicable) as well as this document.

(4) Each employee will be familiar with the following specific warnings concerning IS security:

(a) Do not share access/verify codes with anyone and do not permit anyone to use a system under your authorization code. Do not leave the terminal or microcomputer on-line when unattended.

(b) Do not display or write access/verify codes.

(c) Do not smoke, eat, or drink near the IS equipment.

(d) Do not use IS equipment for unauthorized business.

(e) Label and secure sensitive data printouts and media.

(f) Do not copy copyrighted software packages and do not use copies someone else has made.

e. Physical Security:

(1) The ASLP administrator will ensure that appropriate measures are developed to ensure the protection of IS equipment and peripherals from misuse, theft or unauthorized use.

(2) IS equipment will be located in areas where physical access is controlled, such as an office that can be locked during nonduty hours or in a restricted area. If this is not possible, anchoring devices should be obtained.

f. Sensitive Data:

(1) The ASLP administrator will ensure that all employees are familiar with the sensitive data handled at this medical center and the restrictions on disclosure of sensitive data. The following types of data are considered sensitive in this medical center:

(a) Personal data that identify individuals by name, address, identifying number (SSN), or other specific identifying information, and that includes medical history or diagnosis data, financial transactions, education, criminal history, employment history, and familial relationships.

(b) Resource data pertaining to the control and distribution of funds or diversion of economically valuable assets.

(c) Mission-critical data that, if compromised, could affect the accomplishment of the ASLP mission. Hard copy program listings and associated documentation are considered mission-critical.

(d) Investigative data such as continuous quality management audits, investigations, research studies, and medical center IS audit trails and logs.

(e) Proprietary data used by the ASLP concerning specifications, RFP's, and the award of contracts.

(f) Data, text, and images that are sensitive, but not covered above and that if compromised could result in
misappropriation of funds, fraud, theft, or life threaten-
ing situations.

(2) The ASLP administrator will ensure that all sensitive data
and software media containing sensitive data are kept in a
locked storage area/container when not being used.

g. Back-up of Data:

(1) Data files contained on microcomputers will be backed up.
Backup media will be stored in locked rooms of the ASLP
Service.

h. IS Disaster Contingency Plan:

(1) The ASLP Service will prepare an IS disaster response plan
that covers each IS in the ASLP Service. The ASLP contingency policy will be tested annually.

i. Risk Management:

(1) The ASLP administrator is responsible for the daily over-
sight and supervision of all networked systems to which
the ASLP employees have access.

(2) The ASLP administrator is responsible for invoking discipline or adverse action against its employees for violations
of information security regulations and will ensure that all
suspected or actual security violations are reported to the
medical center's IS officer.

5. References: Medical Center Policy Memorandums:
   Security of Management Information System
   Release of Information
   Security and Control of Medical Records
   Confidentiality of Official Information
   Public Law 100-235, Computer Security Act of 1987
   Public Law 93-579, Privacy Act of 1974

6. Rescissions: None

7. Rescission Date: July 9, 1993

Signature (ASLP Administrator)

APPENDIX 7C

IS Security Agreement and
Computer Access Application—Sample

The following IS security access agreement is adapted from the Audiology and Speech Pathology Service, Veterans Administration Medical Center, Little Rock, Arkansas, submitted by Kenneth W. Heard, PhD.

General IS Agreement
I agree to treat information obtained from computer systems by direct access or by other means confidential.

Computer Access Agreement:
I agree that in the event I am given access to the computer system that it is my responsibility, as a user, to protect my access/verify code from being disclosed to others. I agree not to use someone else's access/verify code.

I also understand that I am being given access to a computer system and that misuse of the system or data contained therein is a criminal offense. Penalties for misuse range from fines up to $5,000 for a first offense minor violation and can be as serious as $50,000 and/or 10 years in prison according to Chief Medical Director's letter, dated June 1, 1993.

EMPLOYEE'S SIGNATURE _____

Employee Name: _____ SSN: _____

Action: [ ] New User [ ] New Access Code [ ] New Menu Only

Mail Code/

Service_____ Division _____

Title _____ Phone _____

Menu_____ Data Base Access_____

Keys_____ Mail Groups_____

Application Coordinator Approval _____

Service Chief _____ Date_____

Chief, IRM _____ Date_____

Approve: [ ] Yes [ ] No

Registered By_____ Date_____

8

FINANCIAL MANAGEMENT

David R. Cunningham, PhD and
N. Rock Erekson, MBA

"All health care managers must be familiar with the financial and productivity aspects of their departmental responsibilities, otherwise someone else will do it for us."

Thorough financial planning and management are essential to the success of any enterprise. Given the fact that ASLP administrators receive limited academic training in working with budgets and in developing profitability targets for their departments, it is unlikely that any manager is skilled in many aspects of these tasks. Program administrators who work in major medical centers or clinics know that these and other important management functions are dispersed among a team of specialists. These experts provide advice in planning new ventures and in solving problems to assure the viability and smooth operation of health care programs.

Even the seasoned administrator must be familiar with the fundamental aspects of financial management and planning. The primary focus of this chapter is to identify and to describe those basic principles that underlie successful business practice. This information will help prepare ASLP administrators in formulating appropriate questions when communicating with advisors to help avoid those common pitfalls that destroy health care practices.

DISCOVERY PHASE

Anyone contemplating the development of a new enterprise would be ill-advised to proceed without expert help. Because good advice from consultants is not usually free, the best way to start is to educate yourself. Invest time before investing money. This self-help phase is a process of discovery. Discovering the issues, trends, strategies, techniques, and philosophies of business management is an essential prerequisite to all that follows. Start with a visit to your library. Read as much material on the topic of management as you can digest. Contact the Small Business Administration (SBA). They will send a bibliography pertaining to business management and finance. Their booklets provide sound, fundamental information written for "lay" managers. The cost for these items is nominal. Attend management seminars offered by professional organizations, local universities, and other consulting groups. Ask state and local governmental agencies for copies of regulations pertaining to facility accreditation, certificate of need procedures (if applicable), tax obligations, business licenses, practice standards, and so forth. Make appointments with representatives of the major third-party payers in your region: Blue Cross/Blue Shield, private health insurers, Medicaid, Medicare, workmens compensation, vocational rehabilitation, and the like. Discover the range of services covered and fees paid in your area of expertise. Learn their methods of payment, whether the payments are fee for service, capitation (a uniform per capita payment or fee), or package priced. Determine their procedure coding and billing mechanisms. This will have a significant effect on how you structure aspects of your practice. Talk to an insurance broker about the kinds and costs of general comprehensive business insurance, personal health insurance options, malpractice liability, employee benefits coverage, long-term disability insurance, and the like. Those readers currently working in an academic setting may find a wealth of information available from colleagues in the school of business. Another good strategy is to visit successful practitioners or clinic directors in geographic regions other than your own (so as not to be viewed as a direct competitor). Ask them how they conduct their business. How are they organized? What advice do they have to offer a novice? Many of these entrepreneurs are proud of their achievements and are eager to share their knowledge.

Most of the preceding advice can be had at relatively low cost. It is now time to carry important questions to those consultants who are going to charge a fee for their services. Two key advisors will be an attorney and an accountant. They will help you understand the myriad of details pertaining to your business organization, day-to-day financial management, planning, tax obligations, personnel issues, liabilities, contracts, and so forth. Find an attorney and accountant who have experience with professional service laws and businesses.

Perhaps the most critical advisor will be the loan officer at the bank or the person(s) who has financial responsibility in the existing organization. Lenders are essentially risk managers. Their job is to weigh the risk to their institution against the probability of your having success. The likelihood of obtaining adequate funding for the enterprise is enhanced considerably by presenting a thorough and realistic business plan for the lender's or financial officer's careful scrutiny.

DEVELOPING A BUSINESS PLAN

A business plan is composed of several components which are essential and necessary. These are: (1) the statement of purpose (mission), (2) justification for the project, (3) proforma profit and loss (P&L) statement, (4) business organization, (5) marketing the program, (6) the business concept, and (7) request for funding.

The authors wish to digress for a moment to discuss a management tool that has proved very useful in their professional setting. It is known as SWOT analysis. The acronym stands for "Strengths, Weaknesses, Opportunities, and Threats." Prior to undertaking a new venture, list as many strengths, weaknesses, opportunities, and threats that may affect a new enterprise as possible. This "brainstorming" strategy helps to define the formal business plan. For example, what are the strongest aspects of the proposal? What are its weaker points? What opportunities can be exploited? What threats might undermine the proposal? Consideration must be given to all facets of the project. Table 8–1 provides an example of the SWOT technique used prior to establishing a hearing aid dispensing unit. The SWOT lists can be expanded as circumstances dictate. This technique identifies those variables that will affect the statement of purpose (mission).

Statement of Purpose (Mission)

The mission component of the business plan should be succinct and represent the program's reason for being in existence. The mission statement (previously discussed in Chapter 2) should answer the following questions:

- ■ What is the program?
- ■ Why does the program exist?
- ■ Whom will the program serve?
- ■ What services will be provided?

Table 8–1. Illustration of the SWOT (strengths, weaknesses, opportunities, and threats) technique.

Strengths:

■ I have 10 years experience.
■ My credentials are superior.
■ I really like amplification technology.
■ I have sufficient cash reserves.
■ Hearing aids are more acceptable to consumers now.

Weaknesses:

■ I have limited business management experience.
■ We are in a recessionary economy.
■ I have no line of credit established with vendors.
■ My energy level is not what it used to be.
■ My site isn't near public transportation lines.

Opportunities:

■ Competition is limited in my region.
■ The elderly population is expanding locally.
■ A prime office site is available near the hospital.
■ I have good rapport with several physicians.
■ Ma & Pa Jones (dispensers) are retiring soon.

Threats:

■ The local otology clinic may begin dispensing soon.
■ I may lose some of my physician referrals.
■ Interest rates are predicted to climb.
■ My sales projections may be too optimistic.
■ The large Acme Manufacturing Plant is closing next year.

For example, "The Suburban ASLP Center is a facility devoted to the diagnosis and treatment of children and adults with communication disorders including speech, language, and hearing impairment. The Center exists for the purpose of reducing the effects of these disorders while enhancing communication skills in patients of all ages. A full spectrum of services will be offered for this population including speech and language evaluations, hearing tests, speech-language therapy, aural rehabilitation, and hearing aids."

Justification for the Project

The justification for the project must answer the question, "Why is this service necessary?" The answer to this question is based on a thorough needs assessment. The intent here is to convince reviewers that a legitimate need exists for new or expanded services. The basis for justifying the need for a new venture may include:

■ *Incidence of the disorder.* What proportion of the general population is likely to have this problem? Is the incidence higher in special subsets of the population to be served (i.e., the aged, the mentally handicapped, etc.)? Are there trends or predictions that can demonstrate the likelihood of increasing need in the future? How many patients will be helped?

■ *Local and regional demographics.* What are the characteristics of the potential pool of customers? Is the population growing or contracting? What is the age, socioeconomic level, and distribution of the patient base? How do the data relate to the specific service(s) provided? Are these patients likely to be able to pay for service(s)? Are they likely to have health insurance or other benefits to cover the cost of service(s)? Is the facility likely to attract patients from a regional geographic area (i.e., a tertiary medical center)?

■ *Competition.* Who are your competitors? What are their characteristics? Will your project provide direct competition or fill a void in the community? What are the unmet needs in service? Can you provide a better service than the competition? What market share will choose your facility?

■ *Inducements.* What referral sources will direct patients to your program? Are there other agencies that will provide assistance? Which are these agencies? What is the probability that these agencies will refer patients? Is this project endorsed by members of the hospital staff, board of directors, and so forth? Has the appropriate funding been promised by the administration, granting agency, or government?

■ *Qualifications.* What are the qualifications of the staff? Are their skills contemporary enough to provide high quality services? How much experience do they have in this particular area of service? Does the practice have sufficient personnel to undertake the project?

■ *Consequences.* What are the negative consequences of not doing the project? For the patients? Institution? Community? Will the competition fill this need if you do not? Are there negative consequences of not being the first to offer this service?

Proforma Profit and Loss (P&L) Statement

The proforma financial projection is the next component of the business plan. The term proforma is Latin for "as a matter of form," and refers to a presentation of data where certain dollar amounts are hypothetical or best estimates. The P&L statement (often referred to as an income statement) is a financial "blueprint." It summarizes all revenues, costs, and expenses of a business during an accounting period, usually one year. The P&L is a standard financial tool used by a business to plan and to communicate to others outside the business (e.g., bankers and accountants). The manager usually provides the accountant with a list of assumptions concerning the program, such as:

- Sales forecast. The projected number of units of service (or number of units sold) on a monthly basis. A unit is defined as a division of quantity accepted as a standard of measurement or of exchange. For example, in the commodities markets, a unit of wheat is a bushel, a unit of coffee a pound, and the unit of U.S. currency is the dollar. In ASLP, a unit estimates how busy the clinic will be each month for the first 48 to 60 months of operation. For example, in the first month, the clinic expects to provide 10 units of service; this will be increased by 4 additional units of service each month through the 24th month of operation. Beginning with the 25th month, 3 additional units per month will be provided.
- The cost per unit or, in the case of products, the cost of goods sold (COGS) represents the wholesale cost of a particular service/product to the program. The COGS will increase over the time frame of the operation and should be commensurate with the Consumer Price Index (CPI). CPI measures the change in consumer prices (e.g., cost of housing, food, transportation, and electricity) as determined by a monthly survey of the U.S. Bureau of Labor Statistics.
- The price per unit represents the charge to the consumer for services/products. This is analogous to the retail price per unit. Prices must be adjusted periodically to reflect increasing costs.
- The fixed cost per month represents items such as lease, rent, utilization fee, utilities, telephone services, insurance, equipment depreciation, and taxes. Fixed costs remain constant regardless of sales volumes. Although no costs are purely "fixed," this assumption serves the purposes of cost accounting for limited planning periods.
- The variable costs per month represents items such as personnel salaries/benefits, custodial services, and marketing expenses. Variable costs change directly with the amount of production (e.g., direct material or direct labor needed to provide services).
- The cost of loans, positive (coming in) and negative (going out), cash flow loans, and so forth.
- One-time (start-up) costs for capital equipment, such as furnishings, instrumentation, durable goods (e.g., photocopiers, fax machines, etc.), and inventory.

An accountant will use these estimates and assumptions to calculate gross profit and net P&L for each month of operation. The ASLP program is expected to show a loss for the beginning months of operation and this must be taken into account when making financing arrangements with a lender (bank). Sufficient funds must be borrowed to cover the losses anticipated in the beginning months of operation. Eventually, a breakeven point (the point at which sales equals costs) is reached. Afterwards, the enterprise should produce a sufficient profit to justify the initial investment of time and money. Profits are used to expand the business or to pay shareholders (when applicable). In either case, the P&L is a standard mechanism to project the growth of a business and to help justify its existence. The lender (or top management) will expect to see the aforementioned documentation included in a business plan. An example of a proforma statement is displayed in Table 8–2. The next component of the business plan includes a brief description of the business organization.

Business Organization

The health care organizational chart shows the position of the ASLP program in relation to other programs within the institution (previously discussed in Chapter 2). If the enterprise is a freestanding clinic, this component of the plan will include a description of the business structure. For example, will the business operate independently, as a partnership, a corporation, a licensed rehabilitation agency, or as a professional service corporation? There are advantages and disadvantages to each type of business organization, such as tax liabilities, personal financial risk, and dissolution (many of these issues were previously discussed in Chapter 3). The advice of an attorney and accountant is crucial in determining which structure meets the needs, and accomplishes the objectives, of the principal owners. These concerns should be resolved long before the business plan is presented.

Marketing the Program

The marketing component of the business plan describes how the department manager intends to promote the program. A description of marketing activities should include a general time frame and an estimate of cost (if any) for each activity. These costs are reflected in the variable expenses section of the P&L. (For a more in-depth discussion on marketing the program, refer to Chapter 9.)

Business Concept

The business concept represents ideas which make the venture unique. A brief review of the justification for starting the business is required. The program administrator must develop a list of goals and measurable objectives to support and complement the mission statement. This outline should prioritize, in a reasonable time frame, short-term, intermediate, and long-term goals that are directed toward the financial growth and quality improvement (QI) of service delivery. (For an in-depth discussion on the topic of QI, refer to Chapter 5.)

For example, one goal may be to bring quality services to the nursing home population in a three county area surrounding the health care organization. The administrator would proceed to contact nursing home administrators to describe the service offerings, determine the number of patients to be served, and discuss contractual obligations between the nursing home

Table 8–2. New Venture Proforma

CASH BUDGET

KEY VARIABLES

				KEY INFLATORS ESTIMATES		
					Labor Increases	CofGS
Min. Required Cash Balance:	$100	Purchases Pattern:		Year 1	0.00%	0.00%
Beginning Cash Balance:	$100	% of Proj. Sales	26.0%	Year 2	4.10%	4.10%
				Year 3	4.10%	4.10%
Collection Pattern:		Payment Pattern:		Year 4	4.10%	4.10%
% Cash Sales	95.0%			Year 5	4.10%	4.10%
% First Month	5.0%	% Cash Payment	0.0%			
% Second Month	0.0%	% Paid 1st Month	100.0%			
% Third Month	0.0%	% Paid 2nd Month	0.0%			
% Allowance for Bad Debts	0.0%	% Paid 3rd Month	0.0%			
	100.0%		100.0%			

ALL OTHER VARIABLES — YEAR 1

	Jan	Feb	Mar	Apr	May	Jun	Jul	Aug	Sep	Oct	Nov	Dec
Units Sold	8	12	16	20	24	28	32	36	40	44	48	52
Price per Unit (avg price for all units)	$718	$718	$718	$718	$718	$718	$718	$718	$718	$718	$718	$718
Sales	$5,744	$8,616	$11,488	$14,360	$17,232	$20,104	$22,976	$25,848	$28,720	$31,592	$34,464	$37,336
Collections:												
Cash Sales	5,457	8,185	10,914	13,642	16,370	19,099	21,827	24,556	27,284	30,012	32,741	35,469
Collections in 1 Month	0	287	431	574	718	862	1,005	1,149	1,292	1,436	1,580	1,723
Collections in 2 Months	0	0	0	0	0	0	0	0	0	0	0	0
Collections in 3 Months	0	0	0	0	0	0	0	0	0	0	0	0
Other Cash Inflows	0	66,750	9,510	8,216	6,809	5,279	3,616	1,807	0	0	0	0
Total Cash Inflows	5,457	75,222	20,854	22,432	23,898	25,240	26,448	27,511	28,576	31,448	34,320	37,192
Purchases	1,493	2,240	2,987	3,734	4,480	5,227	5,974	6,720	7,467	8,214	8,961	9,707
Payment for Purchases:												
% Cash Payment	0	0	0	0	0	0	0	0	0	0	0	0
% Paid 1st Month	0	1,493	2,240	2,987	3,734	4,480	5,227	5,974	6,720	7,467	8,214	8,961
% Paid 2nd Month	0	0	0	0	0	0	0	0	0	0	0	0
% Paid 3rd Month	0	0	0	0	0	0	0	0	0	0	0	0
Total Payments	0	1,493	2,240	2,987	3,734	4,480	5,227	5,974	6,720	7,467	8,214	8,961
Cash Outflows:												28,200
Payments for Purchases	2,000	1,493	2,240	2,987	3,734	4,480	5,227	5,974	6,720	7,467	8,214	8,961
Wages & Salaries	5,667	5,667	5,667	5,667	5,667	5,667	5,667	5,667	5,667	5,667	5,667	5,667
Rent & Leases	1,250	1,250	1,250	1,250	1,250	1,250	1,250	1,250	1,250	1,250	1,250	1,250
Telephone & Utilities	630	380	380	380	380	380	380	380	380	380	380	380
Insurance	60	60	60	60	60	60	60	60	60	60	60	60
Advertising	15,000	1,200	1,200	1,200	1,200	1,200	1,200	1,200	1,200	1,200	1,200	1,200
Maintenance & Repairs	100	100	100	100	100	100	100	100	100	100	100	100
Supplies (office; etc)	300	300	300	300	300	300	300	300	300	300	300	300
Travel & Entertainment	100	100	100	100	100	100	100	100	100	100	100	100
FF&E Lease	0	1,495	1,495	1,495	1,495	1,495	1,495	1,495	1,495	1,495	1,495	1,495
Owner's Withdrawals	0	0	0	0	0	0	0	0	0	0	0	0
Cash Flow Finance – Repay	0	5,837	6,669	7,388	7,983	8,445	8,761	8,919	8,919	8,919	8,919	8,919
Capital Expenditures	47,000	0	0	0	0	0	0	0	0	0	0	0
Other Outflows	100	100	100	100	100	100	100	100	100	100	100	100
Total Cash Outflows	$72,207	$17,982	$19,560	$21,026	$22,368	$23,576	$24,639	$25,544	$26,291	$27,037	$27,784	$28,531
Net Cash Flow	(66,750)	57,240	1,294	1,407	1,530	1,664	1,809	1,967	2,286	4,411	6,536	8,662
Plus Beg. Cash Balance	100	(66,650)	(9,410)	(8,116)	(6,709)	(5,179)	(3,516)	(1,707)	260	2,546	6,957	13,494
Ending Cash Balance	(66,650)	(9,410)	(8,116)	(6,709)	(5,179)	(3,516)	(1,707)	260	2,546	6,957	13,494	22,155
Less Min. Bal. Required	100	100	100	100	100	100	100	100	100	100	100	100
Required Financing	$66,750	$9,510	$8,216	$6,809	$5,279	$3,616	$1,807	$0	$0	$0	$0	$0
Excess Cash	$0	$0	$0	$0	$0	$0	$0	$160	$2,446	$6,857	$13,394	$22,055

---

and the provider. This would lead to an on-site visit to the facility to finalize the contract with an explanation of the provider's standard business practices. A final discussion could focus on implementing a quality assurance program. This approach allows the administrator to develop specific program goals unique to the setting which can be modified periodically to meet the needs of both the practice and the nursing home(s).

Request for Funding

Request for funding (putting money into investments) represents the final component of the business plan. Administrators must justify each element in the request to potential investors or stakeholders such as bankers (this information is reflected in the proforma statement). This justification is prepared by identifying costs attributed to personnel, equipment, marketing, utilities, and so forth. Costs should be considered either as one-time (start-up) or recurring expense. Additionally, the request for funding should include sufficient funding to cover cash flow during the initial (red ink) stages of the new venture. This may involve cash flow projections to pay bills until sufficient revenues are received. Cash flow projections should be estimated on a monthly basis for a minimum of one year. They should include finance charges related to borrowing money. The advising accountant can assist the manager in developing this aspect of the business plan. An example of a request for funding is given in Table 8–3.

The request for funding justifies the project from a financial perspective. It is used to estimate the revenues expected monthly, over the first 48–60 months of the practice. If there is sufficient probability for success, the lender will release the funds to support the venture. However, acceptance rarely occurs on the initial submission; therefore, the manager should anticipate making revisions to the proposal to be considered for approval. Be prepared to rejustify each item in detail in the revised submission.

Beyond this point, it is assumed that adequate funding for the new project is secured. Therefore, the following discussions will reflect the major aspects of ongoing financial management and planning.

SETTING FEES AND DETERMINING PRICES

The manager is usually responsible for setting fees for services (or products for purchase). Consideration must be given to a variety of factors before setting the fee scale. These factors will be examined, in some detail, with the assumption that the enterprise "exists for profit." Attention must be given to the following fee (price) determinants.

Competition

It is reasonable to assume that competition in ASLP exists in most geographic locales. The business plan has identified the competition; now it is time to determine what other agencies charge for similar services. Competition among professionals should keep fees in balance. Care must be exercised in obtaining pricing from a competitor, as the business may face charges of price fixing under federal antitrust laws and there may also be state laws governing such activities. Legal advice should be obtained to determine an appropriate and legal method for obtaining such information. Unless the manager can justify a substantially higher (or lower) fee based on costs for providing services, it is absurd to charge significantly more (or less) than the competition. Indeed, we are likely to see increasing incentives from state and federal governments to publicize fees to increase competition and thereby reduce health care expenditures.

Table 8–3. Request for funding

Start-up Costs	
■ Capital equipment	$56,000
■ Materiels/supplies	7,300
■ Inventory (for resale)	3,500
■ Deposits (telephones, utilities, etc.)	1,200
■ Insurance (general liablility, etc.)	700
■ Other equipment	900
■ Consultant fees	2,100
■ Leasehold improvements (construction & renovation)	6,500
■ Security deposit (two months' rent)	1,800
Startup Costs total	**$80,000**
Annual Recurring Costs	
■ Personnel	
● Clinic Director	$51,000
● Speech-Language Pathologists (3 @ $32,000 each)	96,000
● Audiologist	33,200
● Secretaries (2 @ 19,500 each)	39,000
● Receptionist	16,300
● Personnel benefits calculated at 28% of salaries	65,940
Subtotal Salaries & Benefits	**$301,440**
■ Equipment (repair & maintenance)	6,000
■ Materiels/supplies	5,000
■ Lease/rent	18,000
■ Utilities	2,100
■ Telephones	4,800
■ Travel & education	5,500
■ Finance costs	4,800
■ Cash flow loan payback	12,800
■ Inventory (for resale)	6,500
■ Marketing	5,000
Subtotal	**$70,500**
Grand Total Annual Recurring Costs	**$371,940**

Higher fees may be justified on the basis of demand for services which may be influenced by the business marketing or positioning strategy. Factors to consider in pricing are one's credentials, years of experience, or specific expertise. Lower fees might be justified for certain services that are highly automated and easily delivered to large numbers of patients (i.e., computerized diagnostic or treatment protocols). Furthermore, exclusivity may enter into decisions concerning fees. If an exclusive arrangement can be negotiated with an employer or insurance company in return for significant new volume of services, a lower per-service charge may be appropriate. On the other hand, if the ASLP clinic is the primary provider in a specific locale its services may cost more. In any case, collections must exceed costs. One may ask, how can the clinic best net a profit in a specific area, one penny on one thousand patients or ten dollars on one patient? The answer to the question hinges on the demand for and competition in services in your area.

Usual, Customary, and Reasonable (UCR) Fees

UCR fees are price schedules, prepared by various companies, which represent the average fee charged by health care professionals practicing in a given locale. Gross deviations from UCR fee schedules will attract the attention of payers whether they are insurance companies, vocational rehabilitation agencies, or the patient. Often the reimbursement for ASLP services is based on UCR fees. Because it costs more to provide services in New York City than in Kansas City, significant regional differences in UCR fees should be expected. *Medicare Part B Medical Insurance* (to help pay physicians' bills for services in or out of the hospital, and for other related services) *uses its own fee schedule which is the sum of several complex components.* This method of calculating fee for service is called *Resource Based Relative Value Schedule (RBRVS).* Health care reform may have a significant impact on fee for service pricing of all types; however at this writing, much remains to be seen.

Discounted Fee Structures

In past years, third-party insurers paid in full or a significant proportion (80%) of the fees charged by the practitioner to the insured patient. Those days are history. Employers, seeking lower costs for employee benefits packages, now shop around very carefully for rock bottom, discounted fees for health care services. HMO and PPO programs (previously discussed in Chapter 2) also offer discounted reimbursements to the practitioner in exchange for evaluating and/or treating large volumes of patients (e.g., a trade union group or a large number of insurance subscribers) at a designated facility. This scenario enables the service provider to engage sufficient numbers of patients to offset the dramatic reduction in fees. This method of pricing may be referred to as "package pricing" if dealing with specific services such as audiometry only or, as "capitation" if dealing with a broad range of services. Think of this as a "quantity discount" for services. An ASLP clinic that does not participate in this discounting process can be certain that their competition will. Fees are negotiated on a per capita basis. For example, the employer may have 3,000 employees and will provide incentives for those individuals with a speech, language, or hearing disorder to use a designated facility. The ASLP manager, in turn, agrees to accept 50 cents/month/employee as payment in full for providing services during the following 12 months (e.g., 3,000 employees × 50 cents × 12 months = $18,000/year). The company will pay the provider $18,000 yearly to treat one patient or 1,000 patients. The manager must decide, based on the relative incidence of certain ASLP disorders, whether this arrangement is fiscally sound.

Accepting Assignment

ASLP programs that accept assignment for a patient's bill agree to be reimbursed for what the insurance company allows for that service (and also agree not to bill the patient for the difference between the fee charged and the insurance company's allowance). Consequently, the practitioner agrees to accept full payment provided by the insurer, with the patient paying only a deductible or copay amount. This is similar to the PPO arrangement where the clinic discounts its fees in exchange for a potentially larger patient base of insurance company subscribers. Being a participating provider may be in the clinic's best interest. As in any discounting scheme, the manager must modify revenue expectations with an eye on balancing the budget. This strategy should be considered as a method of obtaining new service volume or securing existing volume in response to competitive pressures.

Contracting with Other Agencies

The manager may find it desirable to contract with other agencies, hospitals, medical specialists, or clinics to provide services. These might include skilled nursing facilities, intermediate-care facilities, group-medical practices, and so forth. Contracted prices can be negotiated on a fee-for-service basis, monthly or annual lump-sum payment, cost-plus pricing, or by-consultation fee. Contracts with other agencies allow the affiliate to bill and collect fees directly from government agencies (i.e., Medicare) or insurance companies, whereas the provider is unable to act as a billing agent for the practice. Hence, there must be a valid contractual arrangement between the two parties.

Cost-Plus Pricing

The price of many clinical services (and prosthetic devices) is regulated by state or federal agencies. This is known as cost-plus pricing. The provider or clinic may charge a fixed rate above their predetermined costs as specified by a formula or some other form of documentation. For example, the Department of Vocational Rehabilitation or the State Crippled Children's Service may pay $150 over the actual wholesale cost of a hearing aid. Providing services to patients referred from state-operated agencies is a matter that must be scrutinized carefully. The manager will have to determine if the clinic can provide high quality services while sustaining the financial viability of the business. By default, when allowances are inadequate, actual costs are shifted to full-pay patients. That is, patients who pay the full fee are essentially subsidizing the costs for medically indigent patients. A decision to continue under these arrangements is as much an ethical/moral issue as it is a financial one.

Setting fees (or establishing prices) is a multi-dimensional task. Projecting revenues under a mixed set of payment schemes and reimbursement rates is very complex. The program administrator must estimate the proportion of patient mix that will be: (1) private full pay; (2) discounted pay; or, (3) medically indigent. There is no magic formula to establish the right patient mix. Nevertheless, it is clear that the manager bears the responsibility for maintaining the viability of the program. This is a fiscal fact of life, which managers cannot ignore.

TRACKING INCOME

Tracking income (or revenues) is a fundamental business process. The manager must know, at any point in time, *the amount of income generated (collections) and the amount of billed products or services (owed to the business), but not yet collected (accounts receivable).* Several characteristics of these revenues must be known in advance, these include:

- *Type of payment.* What proportion of total revenues were in the form of cash, credit card payment, insurance reimbursement, and so forth?
- *Source of payment.* What proportion of total revenues was obtained from health insurance companies, from government agencies, from individuals (private pay), or from contracts?
- *Referral source.* What proportion of income was derived from each referral source (e.g., nursing homes, physicians, agencies, the neonatal ICU, etc.)?
- *By clinician.* What is the amount of income generated by each clinician? Which ones are the most/least productive?
- *Clinic site.* Which clinic sites are the most/least productive?
- *By service.* What is the proportion of revenue generated per procedure? This can be tracked by current procedural terminology (CPT) code (Figure 8–1).

Answers to these questions will alert the manager to the following options: (1) expand or close certain work sites; (2) initiate productivity incentives (bonuses) for some employees; (3) delete selected services or personnel; (4) renegotiate a service contract; and/or, (5) realign key referral sources. It must be understood that knowledge of both the source and amount of revenue represents only one part of the financial picture. The manager must determine the cost associated with each service. These costs are charged to specific sites, individuals, or services in much the same way that the source of revenue is analyzed. For example, the actual costs inherent in providing 1 hour of adult ASLP service in an outpatient clinic may be determined as follows.

Name _____ New Established Chart _____

Insurance_____ MR#_____

Insurance_____ Invoice _____

Clinician_____ Place_____ Date_____

Injury Date/Onset_____ Referring M.D._____ Return Appointment_____

* Code Procedure	Fee	* Code Procedure	Fee	* Code Procedure	Fee

Audiology Office Charge   **Audiology Office Charge**   **Audiology Office Charge**

Code	Procedure	Code	Procedure	Code	Procedure
92507	Cochlear Implant Fitting	92569	AC Reflex Decay	225.1	Acoustic Neuroma
92507	Cochler Implant Rehab	92571	Filtered Speech	351	Facial Paralysis
92516	VII Nerve Study	92572	SSW	380.10	External Otitis
92541	Gaze Nystagmus	92573	Lombard	380.4	Impacted Cerumen
92542	Positional Nystagmus	92574	Swinging Story	381.9	Otitis Media Acute
92543	Calorics	92576	SSI	381.10	SOM Chronic
92544	Optokinetic	92577	Stenger Speech	381.20	Otitis Media Chronic
92545	Tracking	92581	EVR (EEG) Audio	382.30	Choleastoma
92546	Torsion Swing	92582	Conditioning Play Audio	386.01	Menieres Disease Active
92547	Vertical Channel	92583	Select Picture	386.11	Positional Vertigo
92551	AC Screening	92584	ECOG	387.9	Otosclerosis
92553	AC Threshold	92585	BAER	388.12	Noise Induced Loss
92555	SRT	92589	CNS Tests	388.2	Sudden Hearing Loss
92556	SRT & Discrimination	92590	HAE Monaural	388.30	Tinnitus
92557	AC, BC, Speech	92591	HAE Binaural	389.08	BIL Conductive HL
92562	ABLB, MLB	92592	Hacheck Monaural	389.18	BIL Neurosensory HL
92563	Tone Decay	92593	Hacheck Binaural	389.2	Mixed Loss
92564	SISI	92594	HA6500 Manaural	780.4	Dizziness
92565	Stenger Tone	92595	HA6500 Binaural		
92566	Immittance	92596	H. Pros. Eval.		
92567	Tympanogram	92598	Haid Report Writing		
92568	Acoustic Reflex	92599	Unlisted Procedure Earmold		

* Code Procedure	Fee	* Code Procedure	Fee	* Code Procedure	Fee

Speech Pathology Office Charges

Code	Procedure	Code	Procedure	Code	Procedure
43499	Insert Speech Prosthesis	149.0	Neoplasm, Pharynx	478.4	Vocal Cord Polyps
70371	Video Swallow	150.9	Neoplasm, Esophagus	478.5	Vocal Cord Nodule
92506	Speech Evaluation	161.9	Neoplasm, Larynx	478.6	Laryngeal Edema
92507	Speech Therapy	310.0	Cognitive IMP./Head INJ.	784.3	Aphasia
92520	Laryngeal Function Study	331.0	Alzheimer Disease	784.41	Aphonia
		332.0	Parkinson's Disease	784.49	Functional Voice
		335.20	Amyotrophic Lateral Sclerosis	784.49	Hoarseness
		357.0	Guillain-Barre	784.5	Dysphasia/Dysarthrisa
		436.	CVA	784.69	Apraxia
		464.0	Laryngitis, Acute	787.2	Dysphagia
		476.0	Laryngitis, Chronic	854.0	Closed Head Injury
		478.30	Vocal Cord Paralysis		

Previous Balance $_____

Fee $_____

Payment $_____

Balance Fee $_____

Figure 8–1. ASLP computer procedural terminology (CPT) codes.

- ■ Personnel devoted to this activity $15,000/year
- ■ Space (@ $12/sq ft/yr) 7,000/year
- ■ Supplies & materials 1,200/year
- ■ Equipment (maintenance & amortization) 1,800/year
- ■ Telephone & utilities (estimated) 400/year
- ■ General overhead/administration costs 1,000/year

                 Total estimated costs..............$26,400/year

$$\text{Estimated cost/hour} = \frac{\textit{Total} \text{ estimated costs}}{2{,}080 \text{ work hours/year}}$$

$$= \frac{\$26{,}400}{2{,}080 \text{ work hours/year}}$$

$$\text{Estimated cost/hour} = \$12.69$$

Assume that $59,000 was collected (not just billed) under the audiological assessment CPT code (#92557) last year. This represents $28.37 of gross revenue per hour ($59,000/2,080 hr/yr), or about $15.68/hr of net profit ($28.37 − $12.69 = $15.68) derived from this procedure for each hour the clinic is in session. The manager must determine if this particular service offering, and the provider's productivity level, generates sufficient profitability to warrant employee retention or expansion of service. This type of analysis is useful for inspecting the majority of services offered. If a particular procedure is unprofitable, it may be necessary to provide the service to attract patients to other ASLP services. In business parlance, this is referred to as a "loss leader" (i.e., offering a service at a loss, to attract consumers to more profitable services). For example, it may be advantageous to offer screening services at a loss to gain access to a larger population of patients who require other diagnostic or treatment procedures. Similarly, the use of battery clubs can be operated on a break-even basis as a marketing tool to retain customers. Knowledge of the profit margin for each procedure aids the manager in making decisions concerning the assignment of resources and personnel. Remember the business maxim, "No Margin, No Mission."

FINANCIAL REPORTS AND MANAGEMENT INFORMATION

An essential function of the manager is to monitor the financial status of the enterprise. Program administrators must collect, analyze, disseminate, and explain data that accurately reflect the viability of the department and its functions. Relevant information must be obtained on a daily, monthly, and quarterly basis so that comparisons with planned results from previous quarters can be graphed and trended. The information must be accurate, timely, and meaningful. The flow of information must be planned so that these periodic inputs can be interpreted by those individuals who will make decisions and judgments that affect the clinic's operation.

To put the reporting mechanism into proper perspective, the data may not lie but are usually subject to criticism and interpretation. The authors digress a moment to make an important point by analogy. In many ways, financial statistics are analogous to research statistics found in scientific journals. Interpretation of the data is influenced by the statistical analysis methodologies. Financial reporting is no different in this respect. These reports must be interpreted cautiously by the manager and the clinicians who provide professional services. This rationale brings financial data to life in a corporate environment.

In the following sections, the authors will examine several financial/management reports that have proved to be most useful in their professional setting. These reports will be provided along with explanations of their key features. These descriptions are not necessarily presented in order of importance, nor are they by any means exhaustive in scope. It is important to realize that depending on the clinic's particular operation and style, reports other than those discussed may be appropriate in some instances.

The following financial reports are based on the *cash basis of accounting*, the most common method in the health care industry. *Under the cash basis, revenue is measured or assets and liabilities recorded only when cash is received.* Cash transactions referred to include actual cash, cashiers checks, personal checks, credit card receipts, and the like. Charges or billing transactions are noncash transactions recorded on the books of the entity. The manager may encounter the terms "debit" and "credit." Often, a misunderstanding of these terms may cause a manager problems in communicating with those familiar with financial statements. *Debits and credits are accounting terms which very simply describe the location of an amount on a specific account or "T" ledger.* Debits and credits are not necessarily positive and negative numbers *Debits are always on the left, credits always on the right of a specific ledger, such as a patient's account.* Professional assistance should be engaged to structure an accounting system properly from which these several reports may be created. The task of describing all possible working financial reports, their double entry accounting structure, and their variations, however, is beyond the scope of this chapter. The financial reports are often the product of computer software financial management packages. These software programs are commercially available from a variety of sources. Use of these programs should not be divorced from professional review by a certified public accountant (CPA). A CPA can serve a valuable role in properly structuring the financial system of your business. Popular electronic spreadsheets may be valuable in compiling data for management information. Several management software packages are currently available for ASLP application. This information should be apparent from the previous discussion presented in Chapter 7.

Statement of Assets and Liabilities

The statement of assets and liabilities report (also known as a balance sheet) depicts the status of a company's assets, liabilities, and owners' equity on a given date, usually the close of the month or end of the year (Table 8–4). *Assets represent anything tangible having commercial value that is owned by a business.* Usually there are two types of assets, *liquid and fixed. Liquid assets are usually cash or assets which could be quickly turned into cash (e.g., certificates of deposit). Fixed assets often represent tangible property used in the operation of a business.* This property is not expected to be consumed or converted into cash (e.g., equipment, furniture, fixed, and leasehold improvements). Fixed assets are represented on the balance sheet at their net depreciated value. *Depreciation is a noncash accounting procedure that gradually reduces the value of an asset through periodic charges to income.* For fixed assets the term used is depreciation, and for wasting of natural resources the term is depletion. Depreciation is that portion of the cost of an asset charged off to expenses based on a predetermined plan. ASHA (1985) reports several commonly used methods to determine depreciation. These include:

- ■ Offsetting the entire cost as an expense at the time of purchase.
- ■ Estimating the life expectancy of an asset and recording the entire cost as an asset at the time of purchase. Annually, that portion of the asset that loses value is charged off as an expense.
- ■ Establishing a replacement fund as a separate restricted account. The amount is added annually to the equipment replacement fund based on a formula of depreciation, with an allowance for increased costs due to inflation and technological advances.

Table 8–4. Statement of Assets & Liabilities (Balance Sheet) for an Audiology Business as of December 31, 1992 and 1991.

	END OF YEAR	
	1992	1991
ASSETS		
Cash (Liquid assets)	$161,446	$136,292
Equipment (Fixed Assets)	167,101	122,846
Less: Accumulated Depreciation:	7,114	6,566
TOTAL ASSETS	$321,433	$252,572
LIABILITIES		
Payroll withholdings	$2,766	$2,570
Notes payable	100,623	106,725
TOTAL LIABILITIES	$103,389	$109,295
OWNERS EQUITY		
Capital stock	$40,000	$40,000
Retained Earnings	178,044	103,277
Total owners's equity (Net Worth)	$218,044	$143,277
TOTAL LIABILITIES & OWNERS EQUITY	$321,433	$252,572

Net worth is the amount by which assets exceed liabilities. For a corpora-tion, net worth may also be known as stockholders' equity or net assets. Net worth is similar to the equity inherent in home ownership. For example, home equity is essentially the difference between what is owed to the mortgage company and what the house actually sells for on the open market. If a home sells for $185,000, and the mortgage balance is $92,000, the owner's equity is $93,000.

A note of caution is in order. A clinical practice may sell for an amount that greatly exceeds the business' net worth. Therefore, the net worth recorded on the balance sheet alone does not determine the price that another person or group is willing to pay for a practice. A myriad of factors establish the actual value of a business. Not the least of these is referred to as goodwill (intangible asset). *Goodwill relates to the reputation of the practice and the probability that former patients (or referrals) will con-tinue to use the services of the new owner(s) once the enterprise is sold.* Goodwill is also linked to the potential for future growth and expansion of the program under the new owner(s).

Ratio analysis is a financial tool that is commonly used to assist man-agers in interpreting a firm's balance sheet. The ratios imply, quantita-tively, the relationship between various entries listed in financial reports. These ratios can then be compared to figures obtained in prior periods to discover trends and identify peculiarities in the balance sheet. These rela-tionships can be compared to standard ratios in the industry which can be used as a benchmark to estimate financial efficiency and areas of defi-ciency. The financial literature is replete with numerous business formu-las and ratios. For example, a commonly used ratio is the *current ratio. This is a measure of liquidity or how much cash is available to cover liabilities. The calculation is made by dividing current assets by current liabilities.*

A business enterprise can be viewed as a mass of capital (assets) arrayed against the sources of that capital (liabilities and equity), and the balance sheet is a listing of the items making up the two sides of the equation. Unlike a P&L statement, which shows the results of the opera-tion over a period of time, a balance sheet shows the state of affairs at one point in time. A balance sheet must be analyzed and compared to prior balance sheets and other financial reports.

Income Statements

As discussed earlier, income statements summarize the collections and expenses for a specified period. This information is usually reported on a monthly, quarterly, or annual basis depending on the needs of the business. Table 8–5 represents an income report for fiscal years 1992 and 1991. This report is historical and may be compared to the cash budget for planning. This statement may also be used to estimate the next end-ing cash balance. Income reports provide a reference point for decision

Table 8–5. Statement of Revenues Collected and Expenses (P&L) for an Audiology Business as of December 31, 1992 and 1991.

	END OF YEAR	
	1992	1991
REVENUES		
Collection Source 1	$277,220	$116,316
Collection Source 2	246,418	103,392
Collection Source 3	92,407	38,772
Interest	641	717
TOTAL REVENUES COLLECTED	$616,686	$259,197
EXPENSES		
Cost of Goods Sold	$153,451	$59,498
Wages & Salaries	70,788	68,000
Rent & Leases	32,935	31,440
Telephone & Utilites	4,560	4,810
Insurance	720	720
Advertising	61,604	28,200
Maintenance & Repairs	1,200	1,200
Supplies	3,600	3,600
Travel & Entertainment	1,200	1,200
TOTAL EXPENSES	$330,058	$198,668
DISTRIBUTIONS TO OWNER	$100,000	$70,000
EXCESS (DEFICIENCY) OF REVENUE		
COLLECTED OVER EXPENSES AND DISTRIBUTIONS	$186,628	($9,471)

making and allow management to evaluate trends and redirect cash investments or financial outlays.

The income statement adheres to the general format of the P&L statement depicted in the business plan. The difference between these two reports is that the former is based on the best estimates of income and expenses, while the income statement is based on actual figures. The P&L statement becomes a tentative budget or a series of financial targets. During the developmental stage of a new enterprise (i.e., the first 12 months), the manager needs to compare the P&L statement to the actual data depicted in the monthly income report. This comparison will detect errors (over-or-underestimates) in income or expense assumptions, and permits the refinement of the remainder of the P&L statement and budget. Having made these adjustments, the manager can generate a realistic budget for the following calendar (or fiscal) year and beyond. Your banker will be interested in regular updates of the proforma and the actual balance sheet statements. (A fiscal year is an accounting period covering 12 consecutive months at the end of which the books are closed and profit or loss is determined. A company's fiscal year is often, but not necessarily, the same as the calendar year. The fiscal year of the U.S. Government runs from October 1 to September 30.)

Accounts Receivable Report (ARR)

Accounts receivable represents the largest component of working capital and thus requires the manager's concern and attention because it is a key factor in analyzing a company's liquidity. An increase in accounts receivable is viewed as a loss of liquidity; although working capital is unaffected, cash collections may not keep pace with billings for new accounts arising in a given period. A decline reflects an increase in cash collections and is desirable. However, interpretation of ARR is susceptible to misinterpretation due to seasonal fluctuations in billing volume and collection. To be useful, ARR must be compared to other financial reports to avoid these short-term fluctuations. If the manager is to maintain the financial integrity of the program, it is a prerequisite that the accounts receivable collection system operates effectively and efficiently. An example of an accounts receivable report is shown in Table 8–6. There are several accounts receivable reports: charges and collection report, aging report, individual account claim status report, insurance company aging report, payments and collections report, and revenue and production report.

Charges and Collections Report

The charges and collections report depicts the monthly charges and collections for individual (or group) providers within the department. The software programs usually dictate the format for this information; however, Table 8–7 provides an example of information which should be available. Using a cash basis of accounting, a "charge" is a noncash debit to the accounts receivable. This debit is the dollar amount of your UCR for a particular procedure code. A payment or collection is an actual payment received on an account and is credited to the accounts receivable. The format for this type of report again is often dependent on the accounts receivable software used and the level of detail in the set-up. Although the format may vary, there are basic elements of information any such report should contain. This report should provide the source of collections (usually by payer), the detail of adjustments, and the detail of charges by CPT code. There will usually be a recap of all the foregoing detail. This report may be used to provide a basis for several performance measurements.

One measure of the rate of actual cash inflow is use of the average months or days outstanding. This ratio is sometimes referred to as the accounts receivable turnover ratio (ARTO). This ratio is calculated by dividing cash collections for the period (average daily collections or total collections for a month) into the accounts receivable at the end of a month. This ratio gives the man-

Table 8–6. Accounts Receivable Report as of December 31, 1992.*

	January	February	March	April	May	June	July	August	September	October	November	December
Current month billings	$120,000	$120,000	$100,000	$100,000	$100,000	$100,000	$80,000	$100,000	$100,000	$100,000	$100,000	$100,000
Beginning A/R balance	$100,000	$112,050	$109,250	$95,648	$84,648	$75,015	$65,843	$45,092	$47,800	$42,745	$40,355	$33,318
	$220,000	$232,050	$209,250	$195,648	$184,648	$175,015	$145,843	$145,092	$147,800	$142,745	$140,355	$133,318
Cash Received	$106,000	$120,000	$102,000	$102,000	$100,000	$100,000	$94,000	$90,000	$98,000	$98,000	$100,000	$100,000
Adjustments:												
Payment	($50)	($200)	$0	($1,000)	($150)	($60)	($2,000)	$0	($200)	($3,000)	($100)	$0
Charge	$2,000	$3,000	$11,603	$10,000	$9,782	$9,232	$8,751	$7,292	$7,255	$7,390	$7,137	$7,018
Ending accounts receivable balance	$112,050	$109,250	$95,648	$84,648	$75,015	$65,843	$45,092	$47,800	$42,745	$40,355	$33,318	$26,300
Aged accounts receivable												
0 – 30 days	$82,917	$80,845	$70,779	$62,639	$55,511	$48,724	$33,368	$35,372	$31,631	$29,863	$24,655	$19,462
31 – 60 days	$19,049	$18,573	$16,260	$14,390	$12,753	$11,193	$7,666	$8,126	$7,267	$6,860	$5,664	$4,471
61 – 90 days	$10,085	$9,833	$8,608	$7,618	$6,751	$5,926	$4,058	$4,302	$3,847	$3,632	$2,999	$2,367
	$112,050	$109,250	$95,648	$84,648	$75,015	$65,843	$45,092	$47,800	$42,745	$40,355	$33,318	$26,300

* Values are rounded to the nearest dollar.

Table 8–7. Charges & Collections Report.

Time Outstanding	Amount Current Month	Amount Last Month
0–30 days	$71,993	$69,158
31–60 days	$24,831	$23,856
61 – 90 days	$13,016	$12,517
91–120 days	$5,302	$5,108
121–180 days	$2,315	$2,234
Over 180 days	$3,900	$4,067
Total Outstanding	$121,357	$116,940
By Payer		

Percentage of Revenue by Payer	47% Blue Cross		30% Medicare		23% Medicaid	
Time Outstanding	Current	Last	Current	Last	Current	Last
0–30 days	$32,079	$31,144	$24,191	$23,039	$15,724	$14,975
31–60 days	$11,207	$10,881	$7,472	$7,116	$6,152	$5,859
61 – 90 days	$6,529	$6,338	$3,558	$3,389	$2,929	$2,790
91–120 days	$3,169	$3,077	$1,017	$968	$1,116	$1,063
121–180 days	$1,589	$1,543	$286	$272	$440	$419
Over 180 days	$2,764	$2,924	$235	$255	$901	$887
	$57,337	$55,907	$36,759	$35,039	$27,262	$25,993

ager an idea of how long it may take to collect all outstanding accounts receivable at the current rate of collections. The lower this number the less time it should take to collect outstanding bills. This ratio may be plotted by month to build a base of comparative data from which trends may be identified. The turnover ratio is useful because it measures the financial investment that the program has currently in its receivables.

The average days outstanding or turnover ratio is similar to the overall ARR. An increase may reflect a reduction in cash collections and an increased investment in the receivables; a decrease may indicate an increase in payments. The manager may find "smoothing" the plots of data useful to avoid panic in a given month. For example, the average of three months of collections may be used to divide into the accounts receivable to minimize the impact of large monthly increases in charges or collections. The average days outstanding method is also useful in analyzing individual third-party payer accounts. The average days outstanding should be viewed with caution. The write-off policy of the enterprise and the crediting of the aging accounts at the end of an individual period can bias comparative values between different reporting periods.

Another ratio which goes hand in hand with the turnover ratio is the gross-and-net collection ratios. This ratio is calculated by dividing the specified period gross charges (charges before charge adjustments) into the same comparable period gross collections (collections before payment adjustments). This resulting percentage provides a basis of information to determine how efficient the fee structure may be relative to what is actually being paid. A manager may use this method on an individual payer to determine how the fee schedule may be relative to your charges. To achieve a more realistic picture of the overall effectiveness of collection efforts the gross charges should be reduced by charge adjustments (e.g., write-offs or discounts) and the collections changed by the amount of the collection adjustments (e.g., refunds of overpayment):

> **(Collections – Collection Adjustments)/(Charges – Charge Adjustments)**

The closer to unity this ratio becomes, the more effective the collection staff will be at controlling the residual of outstanding receivables. This ratio may be used to determine how effective the billing system is in collecting amounts billed.

Aging Report

The aging report monitors the age of the accounts receivable over time. Usually compiled by the software program or prepared by an auditor, the aging report is a vital tool in analyzing the practices' receivables investment. The report is comprised of a list of receivables by the month, maturity, and extent of delinquency. The aging report shows the balance of a dollar amount since being entered into the billing cycle. The aging report reflects the elapsed time from the date of service to the present. The example given in Table 8–8 indicates that James Doe's balance is $25.00, and that this bill is between 30–60 days old. Julie Done had three separate claims filed with Blue Cross. Claim #20033 is now more than 150 days old; #30666 is more than 30 days old; and #70723 is more than 15 days old. Her total balance is $2,787.42.

We study the aging report very carefully. It provides instant data regarding the balance due, its age, and the status of insurance claims. *The probability of getting paid is inversely proportional to the age of the bill* (i.e., the best likelihood of receiving full payment is on, or near, the date of service). This reality has caused many clinics to ask for payment in full at the time of the visit, and to remit insurance payments to the patient when (and if) the claim is reconciled with the insurer. Obviously, paying in full at the time of service is not feasible in all cases.

The aging report monitors the age mix of the accounts receivable over time. This is established by grouping the individual patient accounts into similar age categories and determining the relationship (in %) of each category to the total accounts receivable outstanding. Interpretation of the aging report facilitates understanding of the effectiveness of credit, payment, and collection policies. An increase in the proportion of new accounts indicates improved cash flow; an increase in the older accounts indicates a reduction in payments. However, like the overall accounts receivable method, the aging report must be interpreted carefully to avoid misinterpretation.

Individual Account Claim Status Report

Closely related to the aging report is the individual account claim report. It depicts the status of insurance claim activity for each individual patient. This is presented in Table 8–9 which indicates that Julie Done has three insurance claims which are in the process of payment. For claim #20033 which was billed on March 2, 1993, the insurance company has paid $749.69 of the $1,000 charge. The insurer actually allowed $937.11 for this service. (Remember: the insurer doesn't necessarily allow as much as the ASLP might have charged). This being the case, the bill was adjusted by $62.89 ($1,000 − 937.11 = $62.89), and the patient was billed for the difference between the allowed amount and actual payment; the balance due is $187.42 ($937.11 − $749.69 = $187.42). The cumulative claims status is shown in the remainder of the data.

Insurance Company Aging Report

Similar in structure to the individual patient aging report, the insurance company aging report indicates the age of third-party balances. Each of the practice's major insurance participants is listed separately along with a monthly account of receivables due the clinic by epoch (i.e., 0–15 days, 15+ days, etc.). The manager can determine not only the total accounts receivable from each insurer, but also the delay experienced in obtaining payment. This format can be used to track receivables from contracted organizations in which the practice participates.

Payments and Collections Report

Receiving prompt and full payment for services rendered creates cash flow that keeps the program in business. Unexpected time delays in receiving payment create a cash flow bind for the enterprise (i.e, expenses increase while waiting for payment). A proper balance between accounts receivable and gross earned revenue will alert the manager that sufficient operating capital is on hand to remain in business. This matter brings up the issue of collections and appropriate mechanisms to receive payment. To achieve that balance, the manager must develop an ethic about the level of aggressiveness with which collections are to be pursued from the insurer and patient. A systematic strategy must be developed for obtaining collections. Fortunately, our group practice has the staff to support this function. The process of collections often begins before the service is actu-

Table 8–8. Aging Report.

Open Insurance Claim Review

			0 – 15 days	over 15	over 20	over 30	over 60	over 90	over 120	over 150	TOTAL DUE
Account:	39599										
Name:	James Doe										
Phone:	399–3944										
	Insurance Company: Prudential										
	Claim #:	3994	$0.00	$0.00	$0.00	$25.00	$0.00	$0.00	$0.00	$0.00	$25.00
	Total Account		$0.00	$0.00	$0.00	$25.00	$0.00	$0.00	$0.00	$0.00	$25.00
Account:	39532										
Name:	Julie Done										
Phone:	398–3324										
	Insurance Company: Blue Cross										
	Claim #:	20033	$0.00	$0.00	$0.00	$0.00	$0.00	$0.00	$0.00	$187.42	$187.42
	Claim #:	30666	$0.00	$0.00	$0.00	$2,000.00	$0.00	$0.00	$0.00	$0.00	$2,000.00
	Claim #:	70723	$0.00	$0.00	$600.00	$0.00	$0.00	$0.00	$0.00	$0.00	$600.00
	Total Account		$0.00	$0.00	$600.00	$2,000.00	$0.00	$0.00	$0.00	$187.42	$2,787.42
TOTAL ALL ACCOUNTS			$0.00	$0.00	$600.00	$2,025.00	$0.00	$0.00	$0.00	$187.42	$2,812.42

Table 8–9. Individual Account Claim Status.

Account	Name	Insurance	Blue Cross	Date Billed	Billed	Date Paid	Paid	Disallowed	Allowed	Adjusted	Balance Due
39532	Julie Done	Insurance:	Blue Cross								
		Claim #:	20033	02–Mar–93	$1,000.00	30–Jul–93	($749.69)	$0.00	$937.11	($62.89)	$187.42
		Claim #:	30666	01–Apr–93	$2,000.00		$0.00	$0.00	$0.00	$0.00	$2,000.00
		Claim #:	70723	16–Apr–93	$600.00		$0.00	$0.00	$0.00	$0.00	$600.00
		Total Account			$3,600.00		($749.69)	$0.00	$937.11	($62.89)	$2,787.42

ally rendered. Proper contract arrangements with a payer—which include clear terms of timing of payment, processing of claims, and resolution of disputes—will be important to any agreement. Our financial counselors help patients discover exactly what their insurance carrier will cover to off-set the patient's financial obligation. The collections process is evident in the clinic with signs posted in the waiting room(s) stating, "Payment Is Expected When Services Are Rendered Unless Other Arrangements Have Been Made." Consideration may be given to providing a nominal discount (1–2%) if the bill is paid at the window, with an explanation that timely payment reduces clerical time and expense. Patients are given the opportunity to pay with credit cards. While this transaction costs the practice a little extra, being paid in full at the time of service counterbalances this effect.

Patients receive statements showing transactions that occur over the preceding months, listing insurance payments, payments from the patient, and current balance. When the insurance claims process is completed, and if payment is past due, a series of telephone calls and letters to the patients follow. The tone of the letters ranges from a gentle reminder to a series of increasingly pointed notifications that past due accounts will be referred to a collections agency. (Appendix 8A provides sample reminder letters for the readers' review.) In our practice, we can (1) arrange for monthly payments (negotiated with the patient by our staff); (2) write off the balance owing; (3) discount the balance; or (4) turn over the account to a collections agency. Patients are encouraged to make small, regular monthly payments instead of referring the account to a collections agency. These agencies charge a fee for acting in our behalf. This charge is in the range of 30–50%. The last resort is to take the patient to court to obtain a judgment which then may be reduced to garnishment or other methods to secure payment. Our experience indicates that it is in the clinic's best interest to negotiate a settlement with the patient to retain as much goodwill as possible. In today's economy, this is especially important since many patients are either losing their jobs or are experiencing reductions in health care benefits.

An estimate of the amount of bad debts should be made periodically to adjust the clinic's accounting records to reflect the manager's judgment of collection probability. Berman, Weeks, and Kukla (1990) offer several methods to estimate the amount of the bad debt.

- ■ Estimate bad debt as a percentage of total revenues for the period.
- ■ Estimate bad debt as a percentage of the revenues from credit sales for the period.
- ■ Adjust the prior period's allowance for bad debts to equal a prescribed percentage of the accounts receivable posted at the end of the reporting period.

The percentage used depends in part upon the entity's success in past collections and on management's judgment of whether that experience will continue. The allowance should be sufficient at all times to absorb the total of all accounts that are suspected to be uncollectible.

We recommend that different percentages be developed for different age groups and types of accounts receivables. The ability to collect on an account and the experience of the practice may be different for each account. Separate estimates add to the accuracy of the overall estimate. An example of estimating doubtful accounts by age category based on the outstanding accounts receivable balance at the end of the period is shown in Table 8–10.

Report of Collections and Charges

The report of collections and charges, sometimes called a revenue and production report (Table 8–11), *is generated each month for the entire practice and for individual providers.* The report is divided into three major sections: the payments and adjustments section, charges, and totals. This report tracks month-to-date (MTD), year-to-date (YTD), and prior year-to-date (PYTD) figures in each of these broad areas. The first section reports payments by source of payment. (Note: the first four lines under service code.) The first line shows payments by check to our bank lock box; the second line shows payments sent by mail to our offices; the third and fourth lines show payments by check and cash, respectively, at the office window, and so forth. The remainder of the payments section displays collections derived from each insurer, from each HMO or PPO, and from other contracts in which we participate. The next two areas are adjustments. Payment adjustments deal with changes in cash. The charge adjustments deal with noncash adjustments to accounts receivable. The charge adjustments display contractual write-offs as well as self-imposed and involuntary adjustments. The term "Proc Count" indicates the numerical tally of a particular procedural code and may be used in

Table 8–10. Estimate of Bad Debt.

Aging Status	Amount	Estimate % Uncollectable	Estimate for Doubtful Accounts
Current	$40,120	1%	$401
0–30 days	$31,873	1%	$319
31–60 days	$24,831	4%	$993
61–90 days	$13,016	7%	$911
91–120 days	$5,302	10%	$530
121–150 days	$2,315	20%	$463
150 + days	$3,900	30%	$1,170
Total	$121,357		$4,787

Table 8–11. Report of Collectons and Charges.

Payments.

Service Code	Payment Description	Month to Date Amount	Proc Count	Year to Date Amount	Proc Count	Prior Year to Date Amount	Proc Count
00001	CHECK PMT LOCK BOX	$2,024.00	16	$7,192.66	33	$2,352.00	20
00005	PMT VIA MAIL	$444.75	3	$956.75	10	$581.75	12
00006	CHECK PMT OFFICE	$1,175.60	3	$1,862.15	6	$5,876.75	12
00007	CASH PMT OFFICE	$49.50	3	$259.50	5	$43.00	4
00011	MEDICARE PMT	$28.53	1	$28.53	1	$22.40	1
00012	MEDICAL ASST PMT	$116.00	7	$144.00	9	$347.00	4
00014	CHAMPUS PMT	$0.00	0	$0.00	0	$972.77	2
00023	BLUE SHIELD PMT	$0.00	0	$43.60	1	$33.00	3
00030	AETNA PMT	$0.00	0	$0.00	0	$59.00	1
00035	COMMERICAL INSURANCE PMT	$19.75	1	$19.75	1	$0.00	0
00050	HEALTH PLAN PMT PPO	$65.00	2	$65.00	2	$0.00	0
00051	HEALTH PMT PPO	$0.00	0	$0.00	0	$92.72	3
00052	BCBS PPO	$9.60	1	$21.60	2	$60.00	1
00056	PRIVATE HEALTHCARE SYSTEMS PMT	$48.75	1	$48.75	1	$0.00	0
00065	PARTNERS SVS PMT	$84.88	3	$109.97	4	$0.00	0
00069	PHYS PLAN (PHP) HMO	$207.00	4	$207.00	4	$0.00	0
00070	HUMANA CARE PLUS	$0.00	0	$0.00	0	$10.00	1
00093	COLL AGENCY PMT	$0.00	0	$135.00	2	$5.00	1
	TOTAL	$4,273.36	45	$11,094.26	81	$10,455.39	65

Payment Adjustments.

00120	REFUND OVERPAYMENT	$0.00	0	$0.00	0	$2,751.00	6
00125	PMT TRANSFER	$0.00	0	$8.00	1	$84.00	2
	TOTAL	$0.00	0	$8.00	1	$2,835.00	8

Charge Adjustments.

00141	MEDICARE ADJUSTMENT	$49.34	1	$49.34	1	($768.00)	0
00142	WELFARE ADJUSTMENT	$137.00	6	$149.00	7	$337.00	5
00143	OUT OF STATE WELFARE ADJUSTMENT	$0.00	0	$0.00	0	$19.00	1
00144	CHAMPUS ADJUSTMENT	$0.00	0	$0.00	0	$439.60	2
00146	REHABILITATION ADJUSTMENT	$0.00	0	$0.00	0	$5.00	1
00153	BLUE SHIELD ADJUSTMENT	$39.00	1	$132.50	4	$0.00	0
00170	AETNA ALLOWANCE	$0.00	0	$0.00	0	$11.00	1
00171	INSURANCE ALLOWANCE	$0.00	0	$120.00	1	$9.50	1
00190	PARTNERS HEALTH DISCOUNT	$71.00	2	$71.00	2	$0.00	0
00191	TEAMCARE ADJUSTMENT	$0.00	0	$0.00	0	$29.37	3
00192	BCBS PPO ADJUSTMENT	$134.00	4	$156.50	5	$100.00	4
00200	PREFERRED OPTIONS ADJ	$0.00	0	$0.00	0	$13.70	1
00201	PPO HOLD	$0.00	0	$0.00	0	$11.91	3
00256	INTEREST FROM CARRIER	$0.01	1	$0.02	2	$0.00	0
00258	CHARGE REDUCTION	$0.00	0	$0.00	0	$2,279.00	4
00260	COURTESY DISCOUNT	$145.00	2	$596.50	3	$350.00	1
00261	PROFESSIONAL DISCOUNT	$0.00	0	$110.00	1	$0.00	0
00263	COLLECTION AGENCY ADJUSTMENT	$0.00	0	$135.00	2	$5.00	1
00266	UNCOLLECTIBLE	$0.00	0	$0.00	0	$51.00	-1
00272	DR W/O BEFORE COLL AGENCY	$0.00	0	$0.00	0	$19.00	1
00276	NON PARTICIPATING ADJ	$0.00	0	$0.00	0	$90.00	1
00277	SMALL BALANCE WRITE OFF	$0.00	0	$10.00	1	$5.00	1
	TOTAL	$575.35	17	$1,529.86	29	$3,007.08	30

(continued)

calculating rough averages. Comparing YTD with PYTD may give some indication of trends or changes in practice or policy by payers.

The second major element of the report lists services performed by ASLP by CPT code, MTD, YTD, and PYTD revenue derived from each service/procedure. These data document the productivity of each clinician, subgroup, or the entity as a whole, and assist the manager (and staff) in determining which services are contributing to profitability (previously discussed in Chapter 6). Along with the insurance company aging report, this report gives the manager vital information concerning which revenues (i.e., an increase in equity arising from operation) are the most or the least productive. The program administrator can use the data to determine which sources are worth developing and which are relatively less important. The information on payments and adjustments is quite valuable when negotiating new contracts, assigning clinical work, and/or when considering the continuance of existing relationships with third-party payers.

Charges.

CPT Code	Procedure Description						
90000	OFFICE VISITS	$0.00	0	$0.00	0	$5.00	1
90600	CONSULTATION LIMITED	$0.00	0	$0.00	0	$30.00	1
90610	CONSULTATION EXTENDED	$0.00	0	$0.00	0	$80.00	1
92512	NASAL FUNCTION STUDIES	$0.00	0	$290.00	2	$0.00	0
92541	SPONTANEOUS NYSTAMUS TEST	$140.00	7	$140.00	7	$0.00	0
92542	POSITIONAL NYSTAMUS TEST	$210.00	7	$210.00	7	$0.00	0
92543	CALORIC VESTIBULER TEST	$780.00	7	$780.00	7	$0.00	0
92544	OPTOKINETIC NYSTAMUS TEST	$20.00	1	$20.00	1	$0.00	0
92545	OSCILLATING TRACKING TEST	$140.00	7	$140.00	7	$0.00	0
92547	VERTICAL ELECTRODES TESTING	$60.00	3	$60.00	3	$0.00	0
92552	PURE TONE AUDIOMTRY, AIR ONLY	$180.00	3	$715.00	13	$123.00	5
92553	PURE TONE AUDIOMTRY, AIR BONE	$0.00	0	$50.00	1	$0.00	0
92555	SPEECH AUDIOMTRY THRESHOLD	$0.00	0	$50.00	2	$0.00	0
92556	SPEECH AUD THRESHOLD & DISCRIM	$0.00	0	$96.00	3	$0.00	0
92557	BASIC COMPREHENSIVE AUDIOMTRY	$870.00	11	$1,970.00	25	$65.00	1
92565	STENGER TEST, PURE TONE	$0.00	0	$0.00	0	$36.00	1
92567	TYMPANOMETRY	$150.00	6	$425.00	17	$82.00	4
92568	ACOUSTIC REFLEX TESTING	$0.00	0	$76.00	2	$0.00	0
92569	ACOUSTIC REFLEX DECAAY TEST	$0.00	0	$26.00	1	$0.00	0
92585	BRAINSTEM EVOKED RESPONSE REC	$0.00	0	$0.00	0	$650.00	2
92590	HEARING AID EXAM, ONE EAR	$700.00	3	$1,500.00	6	$1,400.00	7
92591	HEARING AID EXAM, BOTH EARS	$400.00	1	$1,200.00	3	$1,800.00	5
92592	HEARING AID EXAM, ONE EAR	$135.00	4	$240.00	7	$340.00	10
92593	HEARING AID CHECK, BOTH EARS	$145.00	3	$243.00	8	$380.00	9
92594	ELECTROACOUSTIC EVAL HEAR MONO	$80.00	2	$180.00	4	$410.00	8
92595	ELECTROACOUSTIC EVAL HEAR BIN	$160.00	2	$340.00	1	$320.00	4
92596	EAR PROTECTOR, SINGLE	$0.00	0	$40.00	1	$200.00	6
99070	SPECIAL SUPPLIES	$1,810.00	13	$4,402.75	48	$7,047.88	50
99071	PATIENT EDUCATION MATERIALS	$0.00	0	$0.00	0	$675.00	1
99241	CONSULT.OP.NEW/EST. PT. LEV.1	$30.00	1	$30.00	1	$0.00	0
	TOTAL	$6,010.00	81	$13,223.75	177	$13,643.88	116

Totals.

	GROSS CHARGES	$6,010.00	81	$13,223.75	177	$13,643.88	116
	TOTAL CHARGE ADJUSTMENTS	($575.35)	17	($1,529.86)	29	($3,007.08)	30
	TOTAL NET CHARGES	$5,434.65	98	$11,693.89	206	$10,636.80	146
	GROSS PAYMENTS	($4,273.36)	45	($11,094.26)	81	($10,455.39)	65
	TOTAL PAYMENT ADJUSTMENTS	$0.00	0	$8.00	1	$2,835.00	8
	TOTAL NET PAYMENTS	($4,273.36)	45	($11,086.26)	82	($7,620.39)	73
	TOTAL FOR PROVIDER	$1,161.29	143	$607.63	288	$3,016.41	219

The third major section is the totals area which summarizes all the foregoing detail. These summary data may be plotted by provider on a monthly basis to give the manager useful perspectives about the overall business as well as individual providers.

Based upon these reports, the manager has available the data necessary both to evaluate the overall effectiveness of the entity's billing, credit and collection efforts, and to pinpoint troublesome areas. Using this information, management should be able to assure that accounts receivable remain at acceptable levels.

THE CLINIC (PRACTICE) AS A CONSUMER

Each ASLP practice is both a provider and a consumer of goods and services (previously discussed in Chapter 5). The clinic purchases goods and services from other vendors. Some of these purchases are products for resale (i.e., hearing aids), while others are for the operation of the business (e.g., expendable supplies, janitorial services, legal services, equipment maintenance contracts, employee health insurance premiums, utilities, rent, etc.). The manager must develop a systematic mechanism for monitoring these expenses, commonly referred to as accounts payable (i.e., an obligation to pay an amount to a creditor). This strategy may increase the profit margin by holding costs down. Creative purchasing allows the manager to shop around for the best price for all goods and services used. This extends to costs attributed to personnel, the largest expense item in any budget.

Accounts payable amounts to owing an account to creditors for goods and services. The monthly financial report may list the age and the amount of the original bill, and payments made to each creditor. In some cases, the creditor will offer inducements for receiving payment in full within a specified time frame. This is referred to as "payment terms." Reference may be made in the syntax of 2/10 net 30. This means a 2% discount may be taken if the balance of the invoice is paid within 10 days; but in any case the entire gross invoice is due in 30 days. Some creditors will allow a running balance for recurring orders, while others will offer quantity discounts for bulk purchases. Whatever payment scheme is used, the manager must scrutinize all accounts payable with an eye toward reducing overhead.

An obligation similar to accounts payable is payroll. Payroll is an important and complex area. Employees are the first-line creditor of the business. A prime responsibility for the manager will be to see the employees are paid promptly, accurately, and consistently. Failure to do so can jeopardize the entire practice. This one item on the books is usually the largest single expense. In some states the legal definition of bankruptcy is failure to meet payroll. A decision needs to be made as to whether the service of processing payroll is to be performed in house or by an outside organization. The manager may also choose to lease employees. There are numerous regulations (local, state, and federal) to comply with and professional assistance should be obtained to be certain all the details of this important task are set up and functioning properly. To add to the complexity, legislation for businesses is increasing and also becoming more and more complex, ranging from the phenomenal wave of employee recruitment guidelines to the endless requirements for retirement administration. The manager may choose to "outsource" these services or to have them provided by an organization with considerable experience in this area. A detailed discussion of this issue is beyond the scope of this chapter but should be an area of attention for the manager.

CONCLUSION

Given the foregoing discussion, ASLPs should have a general understanding of the basic financial management responsibilities that face program administrators. This topic fills great volumes and has a nearly limitless scope. To complicate matters further, the very nature of health care finance is undergoing profound changes as we complete the 20th century. For this reason, the task of the manager is all-encompassing. Managers must make a diligent effort to keep abreast of such changes and upgrade their abilities to cope with these complex financial issues. In essence, this brings the manager full circle back to the "discovery phase" described at the beginning of this chapter. The process of discovering new trends and management strategies is never-ending. Only those who are absolutely committed to this challenge will survive and flourish in the future.

REFERENCES

American Speech-Language-Hearing Association. (1985). *Planning and initiating a private practice in audiology and speech-language pathology: Professional practices.* Rockville, MD: Author

Berman, H. J., Weeks, L. E., & Kukla, S. F. (1990). *The financial management of hospitals* (7th ed.). Ann Arbor, MI: Health Administration Press.

Recommended Reading

Cleverley, W. O. (1992). Essentials of healthcare finance. Frederick, MD: Aspen Publishers, Inc.

Ross, A., Williams, S. J., & Schafer, E. L. (1984). *Ambulatory care organization and management.* New York: John Wiley & Sons, Inc.

APPENDIX 8A

Reminder Letter—Sample 1

DATE:

CUSTOMER'S ADDRESS:

BALANCE DUE: $ _____

Dear_____:

We appreciate and understand the fact that some people encounter problems which prevent the prompt payment of their bills.

We would appreciate full payment for the medical care you have received.

If you are unable to remit the total amount due at this time, please contact our business office at (502) 583-8313.

Sincerely,

Payer Relations

Reminder Letter—Sample 2

DATE:

CUSTOMER'S ADDRESS:

BALANCE DUE: $ _____

Dear_____:

Since you have not responded to our previous correspondence, we must now assume you are not concerned with this obligation.

Unless payment of this balance reaches our office within five working days, your account will be referred to the doctor for possible placement with a collection agency.

Sincerely,

Payer Relations

Reminder Letter—Sample 3

DATE:

CUSTOMER'S ADDRESS:

BALANCE DUE: $_____

Dear_____:

We extend the courtesy to our patients of preparing and submitting their insurance forms and extending credit for sixty days. Your prepared claim is ready to forward to your insurance company. However, we are waiting on the assignment/authorization recently mailed to you.

Failure to return this form renders your account due and payable upon receipt.

Respectfully Yours,

Insurance Department

Reminder Letter—Sample 4

DATE:

CUSTOMER'S ADDRESS:

BALANCE DUE: $ _____

Dear_____:

Payment has been received from your insurance company and credited to your account. The balance after the insurance payment is now due from you. Please indicate your method of payment or call our business office at 583-8312 if you have any questions.

Sincerely,

Payer Relations

REMINDER LETTER—SAMPLE 5

DATE:

CUSTOMER'S ADDRESS:

BALANCE DUE: $ _____

Dear_____:

When arranging for your account to be paid in installments, we do request that the agreed amount be paid on a regular monthly schedule.

So that we may continue the payment arrangements, please bring your payment up to date within 10 days or the full balance will be due.

Sincerely,

Payer Relations

9

MARKETING THE PROGRAM

Joan Damsey, MA and
Denise Mill Parker, MBA

"The people who get on in this world are the people who get up and look for the circumstances they want, and, if they can't find them, make them."
(George Bernard Shaw)

*M*arketing encompasses all that is done to promote a business from the moment of conception to the point at which customers buy the products or services and begin to patronize the business on a regular basis. It involves more than the selling, advertising, and image making with which marketing is usually associated (Kotler, 1980). Marketing analyzes opportunities, defines target markets, designs strategies for reaching these markets, and plans advertising and promotional programs for the organization's products or services. A successful marketing plan is generally not the result of individual genius or effort. Rather, it is the result of the efforts and intellects of a group of individuals who must function together. Program administrators must assure that all marketing efforts will be coordinated and controlled in order to achieve the objectives of the program.

The established patterns and guiding principles of marketing discussed in this chapter are practical and can be applied to almost any situation. The purpose of this chapter is to describe the marketing process and to relate a specific plan to ASLP practice. Admittedly, this plan will not be ideally applicable in all situations. However, it will provide the basis for marketing any entity and should be understood if the reader is to obtain a working knowledge of marketing.

STEP 1: ESTABLISHING THE MARKETING MISSION

For the ASLP program, the marketing mission can be viewed as the broad definition of the scope and purpose of the entire organization. For example, the mission may be to receive referrals from physicians inside and outside of the health care organization, or to support their practices in the multispecialty facility. Large programs, comprised of multiple specialties (see Figure 2–2) may have several mission statements. Although the mission for the entire program remains the same, the scope and purpose of each specialty unit may be quite different. However, each of these separate missions must support and promote the overall mission.

Each program unit has a unique customer population requiring its own marketing and business plans. For example, the marketing plan for a geriatric ASLP unit focuses on senior citizens, while that of a pediatric ASLP unit is likely to be women of child-bearing age. Despite these differences, specialty units must coordinate their marketing activities as much as possible. It is important that each specialty understand the overall mission of the entire program, and the mission, business goals, and marketing plan of each individual unit as it relates to the overall mission. To illustrate, the mission of a hearing aid program must be consistent with the mission of the entire program. It is essential for audiologists to understand the mission of the program, the mission of the hearing aid program, and the hearing aid program's marketing plan. The mission of the hearing aid program may be to provide convenient and affordable access to amplification devices for all hearing-impaired patients within a defined market segment, such as a market defined by location and income. If the hearing aid program is investor owned, a major goal may be to realize a 10% return on investment since stockholders seek a prospectus that indicates an adequate return. Moreover, while the hearing aid program may be required to achieve a 10% return on investment, the entire program may be expected to post a 35% return on investment. Thus, the mission of the hearing aid program is to post a 10% return on investment, while providing convenience and affordability for the patient. Once the mission has been defined, the situation in which the program finds itself is analyzed, and needs are defined so as to make it possible to achieve the mission.

STEP 2: ENVIRONMENTAL ASSESSMENT

The purpose of assessing the environment is to ensure that the program has considered the major factors, both internal and external, that currently affect, or may in the future affect, its operations or performance. The assessment process attempts to gather and analyze information pertaining to present and potential customers, the competition, internal strengths and weaknesses, external opportunities and threats, technology, trends within the profession, government regulation, and reimbursement issues (Kotler, 1980).

Market Segmentation

If the ASLP marketing plan is to be successful, target markets, both internal and external to the organization, must be identified (Weiss, 1990). To identify your current markets, analyze your customer base to see whom you spend the most time trying to satisfy. Review of billing files, medical records, and program reports will also help to reveal the actual markets served. To identify potential markets, decide whom you would like to be serving.

To serve these markets, ASLP administrators must have an understanding of their communication needs and the unique factors that determine each particular population's demand for services (Abell & Hammond, 1979; Hunter, 1987; McDevitt, 1987; Nichols, 1986). The segmentation characteristics of greatest importance in assessing your target market's demand for services and communication needs include population size and rate of growth; age and sex distribution; racial, ethnic, and religious composition; cultural characteristics; income; reimbursement; occupation; education; mobility; and health status. The principal benefit of this target market analysis is in allowing the program administrator to determine existing attitudes toward the products and services offered and to locate potential target markets. The importance of this process of segmenting and targeting markets is to forecast the future size and attractiveness of various current and potential market segments.

A market segment often overlooked is that of referral sources. Their importance should not be underestimated in view of their ability to provide patients, and thus income, to the program. Focusing marketing planning on health care professionals requires knowledge of such factors as their age, specialty, type of practice (e.g., individual, group, etc.), years in practice, and share of total referrals sent by this particular physician (Figure 9–1). In addition to having knowledge about your referral sources, it is important

KNOW THE REFERRAL SOURCE

NAME _____ DATE OF BIRTH _____

TELEPHONE (O) _____ (H) _____

ADDRESS (O) _____

(H) _____

EDUCATION _____

COLLEGE _____

POSTGRADUATE _____

MEDICAL SCHOOL _____

SPECIALTY _____

TYPE OF PRACTICE _____

YEARS IN BUSINESS/ON STAFF _____

HOBBIES and RECREATIONAL ACTIVITIES _____

MARITAL STATUS _____ SPOUSE _____

CHILDREN _____

DINING PREFERENCES _____

NUMBER OF REFERRALS DURING A SPECIFIC PERIOD _____

DOLLARS BILLED _____

SHARE OF TOTAL REFERRALS _____

_____

Figure 9–1. Information sheet maintained on each referral source.

that you ensure their satisfaction with your organization. Send each referral source a copy of the diagnosis, treatment recommendations, and the plan of treatment for each of his/her patients. If the referral source is a current patient, send a personal letter of thanks. Make mention in the letter of how appreciated the referral is, and that you consider it a compliment when a satisfied patient sends a friend or family member to you.

Without knowledge of the target markets, their present and potential need for ASLP services, and their expected rate of growth, the market planning process is irrelevant. Each customer segment is unique with regard to its needs for services, products, and information. To effectively market an ASLP program, you must understand the customer, regardless of how customer is defined, so well that the products and services seem to sell themselves.

Know Your Competition

Knowing the competition requires an assessment of your competitors' strengths, weaknesses, capabilities, and strategic plan for the future. Questions to be addressed include: Who are your competitors? What is the competitive advantage of each competitor? Which competitors are likely to emerge? Where are your competitors most vulnerable? What is each competitor's market share? A practical approach to assessing a competitor is to contact organizations such as:

- The American Speech-Language-Hearing Association
- State Audiology and Speech-Language Pathology Associations
- State Hearing Aid Societies
- State Licensure Agencies
- State Certification of Need Agencies
- Chamber of Commerce
- Bureau of Census

The information obtained from these organizations can reveal much about the competition (Figure 9–2).

A second means of gathering information about the competition is to ask those who know them, such as referral sources, patients, suppliers, and others. Many times, competitors will share information about their practices, if asked directly. It is very important to know what the competitors' patients and referral sources like or dislike about them. Having this information can help you position your service better for your target market.

Internal Environment Assessment

The internal environment of the ASLP program consists of the governing board of the health care organization, the clinical staff, management staff, the office employees, the products and services offered, price issues, distribution/location issues, and promotion issues. *The purpose of the internal environment assessment is to determine where the entity is at the present time.* This must be done before determining where the program is headed in the future. All programs must perform an in-depth evaluation of their strengths and weaknesses, competitive advantage(s), staff capabilities, technology, utilization trends, financial trends, and reputation. This is necessary for effective marketing planning.

Based upon this assessment of the internal environment, service quality should be improved to increase customer satisfaction, volume,

KNOW THE COMPETITION

Part 1. Competitor Profile:

A. Name of Competitor _____

B. Type of Organization/Practice _____

C. Years in Practice _____

D. Size/Volume of Practice _____

E. Competitive Strength _____

_____

F. Competitive Weaknesses _____

G. Probable Competitive Direction _____

_____

H. Probable Long-Term Strategy _____

_____

Part 2. Market Share Profile:

Target Market	Year	Market Share Percent/Percent Change
1.		
2.		
3.		
4.		

Figure 9–2. ASLP competitor profile.

and revenue. Assessment of internal strengths may lead to the development of new services or to improvement of those aspects of the practice needing enhancement. Likewise, assessment of service weaknesses can result in better problem-solving strategies in responding to the demands of the market. Internal environment assessment demands honesty and time by both the ASLP program administrator and the clinical staff. While familiarity may not breed contempt, it may breed myopia. Those aspects of the program which have become routine are often simply accepted without recognition of the aspect's contribution to or detraction from the program. Such small details as proximity to parking or mass transportation can be significant strengths when marketing is directed to senior citizens or parents of small children. But this type of information may go unnoticed without a concerted effort to examine all aspects of the program.

Staff preferences and experience also contribute to the organization's strengths and weaknesses: a staff comprised of individuals with keen interests in adult disorders will be more likely to support marketing targeted to that area. They are also more likely to have the training and experience necessary to allow the ASLP program to promote itself as unusually qualified in the area of adult disorders. Conversely, these same preferences and levels of training and experience impose limitations on the program's ability to expand in the area of disorders found in the pediatric population. Clear comprehension of the program's strengths and weaknesses permits the administrator to establish realistic marketing goals and to promote the program in an increasingly competitive marketplace.

External Environment Assessment

ASLP programs serve many publics: local schools, political organizations, senior citizen groups, medical groups, and others unique to each community. As a result, they are constantly affected by increasing pressures from other disciplines and from business. As payers, businesses are, in effect, consumers of care and certainly feel the major impact of cost increases. In an effort to reduce the cost of health care, competition is increasing, with a resulting reduction in utilization of any single provider, and thus, revenues.

In addition to other disciplines and business, organizations such as ASHA and JCAHO are placing pressure on clinical programs with respect to professional issues such as accreditation, credentials, quality of care, and reductions in university enrollments. Each ASLP program should assess how these organizations are affecting the practice. In addition, evaluate technological developments in the field which, if implemented, could give your practice a competitive advantage. Are there declining or no longer needed services which should be eliminated to transfer resources to more promising opportunities? Assessing issues such as these will help to determine whether the current marketing plan is likely to be successful.

This external environment analysis will lead to a marketing campaign by which program administrators define the program's competitive position through managed combinations of products and services.

Government Regulation

Regulations often vary by program, and several specific regulatory questions should be posed for the major services areas, such as: What kinds of local, state, federal, and self-regulatory controls affect the provision of ASLP services? Conversations with state and national professional associations, politicians, and their staff members are vital to the overall effectiveness of the program's marketing planning process.

STEP 3: MARKETING GOALS AND OBJECTIVES

The purpose of Step 3 in the development of a marketing plan is to put the marketing analysis into an action plan with clear objectives for the next period, usually one year.

Goals define where the organization should go in general terms, while objectives are short-range targets that are measurable in specific terms. Marketing objectives include a measurable outcome, such as units sold, market share, net income, or profit. They should be developed for a specific time frame. Above all, objectives must be realistic. For example, the established organization will be much more likely to effect a 5% increase in patient visits through marketing over a one year period than to increase patient visits by 40% over the same period. An objective answers the questions: What will be accomplished? By whom? And when (date)? Keep in mind that objectives may be related to new service development, existing service development, and/or customer satisfaction.

STEP 4: MARKETING STRATEGY

Marketing strategies represent the broad approach to be used by the ASLP program to achieve its marketing objectives. This includes the selection of markets to be targeted, the choice of a competitive position, the development of an effective marketing mix to reach the target market, and the establishment of a marketing budget.

Market Positioning

The basis on which ASLP providers compete is known as positioning (Aaker & Shansby, 1982). A program seeks to have a market position that is distinct and positive in the minds of its present and potential consumers. Positioning means determining exactly what niche your offering is intended to fill. This is accomplished by analyzing a market segment and then selecting, developing, and communicating the most desirable positioning concept for that particular audience. Health care providers can build a competitive advantage (Jensen, 1986) using a combination of three basic strategies:

- Offering the lowest cost.
- Creating uniqueness through technology, staff, services or quality of care.
- Concentrating on a particular market segment.

Program administrators seeking to position their programs should ask themselves:

- What does this organization stand for?
- What are the objectives of our marketing plan?

- What are our strengths and weaknesses?
- What type of client mix is desired?
- What type of service should we focus on?
- What is our competition doing?

Answers to such questions will lead to the development of a market position that maximizes the organization's strengths and minimizes its weaknesses. Positioning is a long-term strategy which, once firmly established, is difficult to change. The biggest problem is determining which position you currently own and which one you want to own. It is impossible to be all things to all people, making it imperative for the organization to identify its particular target market(s). Organizations which become good at serving the needs of a particular market segment are the ones which prosper.

Realistically, it is difficult for an ASLP program, hospital-based or private practice, to perform much differently from its competition. For example, let's assume that five programs existing in a given locale offer the same services, and their business is down by 10%. Unless a new specialty is developed or a new market segment found, it is unreasonable to assume one program can outperform another in terms of the basic assessment or therapeutic services offered. With four other programs in close proximity, the ASLP administrator probably has little flexibility in pricing without reducing profitability further. Flexibility in scheduling may be possible as a means of attracting more clientele. The administrator may also elect to focus marketing on that portion of the potential market most able to afford the program's services, as this would increase net receipts and improve profitability. Other solutions based on cost, uniqueness, and market segmentation are possible; all require preparation by the administrator. When studying the marketplace, it is important to be compared to similar competitors. This approach will assist the program administrator in positioning the program based on the marketing mix.

The two following examples focus on strategies used to position an organization in the market place.

Positioning a New Program

The development and implementation of an ASLP program in an area with few (or no) competitors allows the program administrator to strive for strong marketplace recognition from the outset. In this instance, strong recognition is associated with being first in the marketplace. The lack of competition and the need to recover start-up costs allows the new program to charge a premium price for its products and services.

A high price strategy can also be used to offset an excessive demand for services by ensuring that demand remains within the program's patient scheduling capacity. However, the quickest way to encourage competitors to enter the market is to set a high price. Potential competitors may feel that they can offer the same service at a lower price while achieving a reasonable return on their investment. The major risk associated with this strategy is dependent on the organization's understanding of its cost and demand curves. Costs must be covered by charges, and demand should not be allowed to exceed capacity. Customer dissatisfaction will result from excessive waits for an appointment or delays in being seen by the clinician. The critical perspective here is not how "reasonable" the delay may seem to program staff, as how unreasonable and presumptuous it may seem to the customer.

Finally, the introduction of a new service into the market place requires the commitment of financial and personnel resources to advertising and public relations. Consumers must be educated about the organization's products and services and their unique benefits before they will seek out the organization. Print and broadcast media advertising, public relations, and personal selling are means of achieving marketplace recognition for a new program.

Positioning an Existing Program

Established programs will experience fluctuation in daily, monthly, or annual patient census. The tendency is to view such fluctuations as "seasonal" or random. The effective administrator, however, should question the fluctuations in the context of both past fluctuations in the patient census and the program's marketing plan. There are two basic strategies to follow in order to level the fluctuations:

- Segment the market by concentrating on the more profitable groups, and attempt to strengthen market share within these segments; and/or,
- Develop new service offerings.

ASLP programs not at the forefront of the offerings of the marketplace should determine if there is some segment of the market that is not being served. Can the service be improved? Can the products or services be offered at a lower price? Should a dynamic advertising campaign be mounted? Increased sales and market share can come only at the expense of a competitor. Thus, the search for new alternatives becomes the only course for growth of an established program. By reexamining the service, the manager can open new windows of opportunity to regain inactive customers or to reposition the service against the competition. One alternative is to reduce the price of the organization's services to keep loyal customers and to attract new customers away from competitors. However, the program administrator should recognize the very real hazards of a price war.

Established ASLP programs must make ongoing efforts to ensure that patients return to them and referral sources continue to send patients to their program. Post-treatment follow-up through letters, telephone calls, or sales force contact is necessary to ensure the continuing satisfaction of the customer, whether patient or physician. Such activities as newsletters and inservice education seminars also become important in keeping a loyal base of existing customers.

Marketing Mix

The marketing mix represents the set of controllable variables used to pursue the ASLP program's marketing objectives (Kotler, 1980). Typically referred to as the "4 Ps of marketing," the primary variables of the marketing mix are product/service, price, place/distribution, and promotion. These variables answer the question, "How should products or services be configured so that they offer customers the greatest satisfaction?"

Product/Service Decisions

The able administrator does not view a product or service as a single entity, but as a composite of a variety of features. These individual features directly or indirectly affect the marketability of the products or services. For the ASLP program, these product/service features include general and specialized services, the skill level of the staff, physical environment, technology, and level of customer service. As the marketing plan is developed the following questions should be answered:

- What are the program's products and services, past, present, and anticipated?
- Are the program's products and services superior to or uniquely different than those of the competition?
- What are the strengths and weaknesses of the current mix of products and services?
- Should any products or services be phased out or added?
- What services are most heavily used?
- What is the financial status of the program's major products and services?
- What are the features of the program that give it an advantage over its competitors?
- What products and services are desired by the target market?

By answering these questions, the program administrator can identify the benefits of the product or service that are basic for successful competition, the benefits offered by each specialty, the specialties which are most competitive, and the options available for redefining the product or service through an alternative combination of benefits.

Pricing Decisions

When making pricing decisions, the program administrator should consider both monetary and nonmonetary costs. The primary nonmonetary costs are the time spent acquiring the service and the time away from work or family. Often, these nonmonetary costs are of more concern to the patient than are the monetary costs. For the customer to be satisfied, the nonmonetary costs must be offset by equivalent service values.

Some program administrators continue to believe that pricing strategies do not apply to health care providers. However, the price set for each product or service should properly reflect the direct and indirect costs for producing the services rendered, plus a reasonable premium for community costs. In other words, the price set should include a cost premium for services provided to the community such as education, research, and ASLP health programs. Most of today's hospital-based ASLP programs are not managed as competitive, profit-making institutions, but instead depend on third parties for reimbursement. What is a third party? It is any agent other than the patient who contracts to pay all or part of the ASLP program charge for services rendered. Although there is a multitude of third-party payers, they fall into essentially three groups: the commercial insurance companies (e.g., Blue Cross/Blue Shield), government agencies (e.g., Medicare, Medicaid, Workers' Compensation), and managed care plans (e.g., HMOs, PPOs, etc.).

Managed care plans appear to be gaining strength as an important factor in the health care marketing environment. As ASLP programs become more competitive, HMOs, PPOs, and other third-party payers will be increasingly price sensitive. In addition, as a cost control measure, most employers are adding significant copayments (as much as 30%) to each health care encounter between a patient and a provider. Such copayments increase patient awareness of price and value. A common characteristic of managed care plans is the emphasis on price competition. As reimbursement changes, it is increasingly appropriate to consider various pricing options. Consider the factors that determine the price of a product or service-cost, competition, demand, and the willingness of third-party payers to reimburse the provider when evaluating various pricing options.

Further questions to ask when determining pricing include:

■ Is pricing based on cost plus, return on investment, stabilization, or demand?

■ How are prices for services determined? How often are prices reviewed?

■ What factors contribute to a price increase or decrease?

■ What were the price patterns in past years?

■ How are the program's pricing policies viewed by patients, referral sources, competitors, and third-party payers?

■ How are price promotions used?

■ What would be the impact of a higher or lower price on demand?

ASLP management must carefully evaluate the pricing alternatives available for meeting the program's goals, and eliminate those which are impractical. The pricing alternatives that might be employed by the ASLP program in pursuing its marketing goals are summarized below.

■ Cost-oriented pricing involves setting a price which allows the organization to recover the costs of program development and implementation. The disadvantage of a cost-oriented pricing is that it often encourages competitors to enter the market.

■ Competitive-oriented pricing involves setting a price at or below the prevailing level in order to compete in the market, or to increase market share. For example, a program may decide to compete in the hearing aid market with a low-cost program.

■ Demand-oriented pricing estimates how much value the customer sees in the product or service and sets prices accordingly. The price reflects the perceived value of the product in the buyer's mind. In this instance, a premium price can be used to develop a status position for the service in the consumer's mind. Buyers are likely to gravitate toward the more expensive program, which is perceived to be better.

■ Maximum-reimbursement oriented pricing entails charging the maximum amount allowed by reimbursement agencies. Depending upon the type of reimbursement available, the ASLP program may have little choice in setting its fees. In some instances, health care fees are regulated by state-mandated rate-setting programs. Or they may result from a negotiated settlement with Blue Cross or other insurers. For HMO and PPO patients, reimbursement is determined by preestablished competitive negotiations between insurers and employers. Thus, the reimbursement categories of the program's target markets must be considered in pricing decisions.

■ Package-oriented pricing charges a "package" price that is lower than the total price for the individual services. Consumers are inclined to purchase such a package when they sense that they are getting a substantial discount (e.g., an industrial hearing conservation program).

Various market segments will respond differently to price changes. For example, many buyers will be attracted to the higher-priced option, believing that high prices mean better service and better quality care. As a result, program administrators who consider price changes must be sensitive to the reactions of their target markets. Moreover, the price structure should be equitable to all parties.

The changing face of reimbursement and competitive trends require close scrutiny of pricing practices. Internally, the rationale for existing prices should be reviewed in the context of external pricing trends. To this end, pricing decisions should be analyzed and justified for each specialty unit within the ASLP program.

Place (Distribution) Decisions

Place decisions determine the manner in which products and/or services are made available in time and space so that customer access is optimized. Physical access and time access are the major place decisions to be made. Physical access to the organization, its location and layout, is critical to its success. Site location, the architectural design, and interior decorating are identified links to the market as well as opportunities to influence the customer. Customer travel time, comfort, and convenience have often determined a health care facility's success. As competition for patients increases, customer preference should determine the site of the facility.

Equally important as physical access is time access. The hours/days of operation must be set to accommodate the target market's needs. For example, consumers who work full-time during normal business hours may desire evening, early morning, or Saturday appointments. In addition, the length of time between calling for and receiving an appointment, and the length of time spent waiting in the reception area to see the clinician, should be kept to a minimum.

Promotion Decisions

Promotion decisions (the final marketing mix decision to be made) outline the manner in which the product/service benefits will be communicated to customers. Resources must be allocated across the most effective communication method(s) for the target market under consideration. The communication methods to be considered include advertising, public relations, and personal selling.

Advertising

Advertising must be tested to ensure that it is understood by the market segments you hope to reach, such as consumers and physicians (MacStravic, 1988). It is important to design broadcast and print advertisements for the intended audience. For example, materials for the general public should be less technical than those designed for medical referral sources. Promotional products directed at senior citizens should not be associated with aging or sensory deficits, otherwise they will be ignored. In any advertisement, emphasis should be placed on your competitive advantage(s). The effectiveness of the advertising campaign should be assessed at the time the customer visits the program. A patient survey asking how and why the particular facility was selected is easy, efficient, and informational.

The majority of programs rarely resort to minimal marketing methods such as canvassing, writing personal letters, telemarketing, distributing circulars, posting signs on bulletin boards, and Yellow Pages advertising. As a result, there will be little competition in these areas should you choose to use them. Regardless of which marketing techniques are selected, they must support the marketing plan. The selection of appropriate methods for advertising your program requires a knowledge of the viewership and even the travel patterns of the target audience. Utilize as many media as your budget will allow, but do not spread the advertising too thin, as it will be ineffective. Use of these advertising media will rarely put a strain on the marketing budget; production cost will be low.

Maximum advertising refers to advertising in newspapers, magazines, on radio and television, and by direct mail. Mistakes cost dearly in these media. The reader should not think of maximum advertising as expensive. Instead, expensive advertising is advertising that does not work. For example, a spot on a local radio station may cost $20, but if no one hears or acts on the information, the program administrator has engaged in expensive marketing. But if $500 is budgeted to run a one day ad on a major metropolitan radio station or on cable television and a $2,000 increase in profit is realized the following month, the cost for marketing is inexpensive. Cost is clearly secondary to effectiveness.

An alternative to the broadcast media are the print media, such as newspapers and magazines. Newspapers offer a high degree of flexibility because ads can be altered until a few days before being printed. The advantage of newspaper advertising is coverage. The vast majority of adults report reading a newspaper at least once a week. Advertisements should be placed in the most appropriate local newspaper, given the audience you intend to reach. If there is a number of newspapers in the region, ads should be placed in as many periodicals as reach your target market. Offering discounts or free services in advertising may be effective, depending upon the area and competition. The major disadvantage of newspaper advertising is a lack of audience selectivity. Many large newspapers have added zip code editions, but these are primarily in metropolitan areas. Consequently, when a metropolitan program runs an advertisement for its ASLP program, it is seen by many readers other than the target market. If the program is not intended for a particular audience, the program has paid for wasted coverage.

Of the advertising media available to the health care organization, direct mail provides maximum audience selectivity and cost effectiveness. Direct mail marketing refers to direct mail, mail order, telemarketing, or any method of marketing directed at a specific consumer which attempts to prompt the consumer to make an immediate decision to purchase the product or service. For instance, if a program decides to target hearing-impaired individuals who are 60 years of age or older, a direct mail house can produce mailing labels for the target audience so that a brochure on the hearing aid program can be sent to a specific audience in the desired market area. This method of advertising ensures a higher selectivity of the audience being targeted.

An advertising checklist may be helpful in making advertising decisions, and should consider the following questions:

- What specific aspect of the program's products and services should be advertised?
- Should the advertising offer a price discount?
- Which competitive advantage(s) should be promoted in the advertising?
- Which target markets does the organization want to attract? Where are they located, and what is the likelihood that they will use the program?
- What principal benefit is the target audience seeking?
- What are the technical advantages of the product?
- Which advertising medium should be used? Why?
- Will the advertisement capture the attention of the desired audience?
- Is the completed advertisement easily read and understood by the target market?

Honest answers to these questions can prove invaluable to the advertising effort. Incomplete answers, or no answers, can prove disastrous.

Public Relations

Public relations means exactly what it says. But it is also accurate to say that it means publicity such as, free news of the organization or staff in newspapers, magazines, newsletters, on radio or television, speaker placement bureau, special events such as health fairs and open houses, and in any other type of media. The advantage to the program is that public relations efforts are free. Public relations are credible and help establish the identity of the organization.

The most overlooked promotional techniques in health care are community organizations, speakers' bureau placement, and networking. Community organizing may take the form of sponsoring a community health fair. Speakers' bureau placement, providing speakers free of charge to interested groups in the community, is a very effective means of promoting an organization, as is networking. Membership in professional societies, participation in outside workshops and conferences, attendance at conventions, continuing education courses related to the ASLP field, research, and publication on related topics serve to promote the program.

Personal Selling

Personal selling is the personal presentation of information to a prospective consumer or group of consumers for the purpose of making a sale or building good will (Kotler, 1980). The overall image created by the clinician and support staff is the single most important personal selling activity. Personal selling should be directed at every audience which may be attracted to the practice. It is an aspect of promotion that most clinicians still do not fully appreciate or utilize to their best advantage.

One means of personal selling to be considered is to establish a small sales force to call on local companies. The purpose of the sales call is to obtain information about the organization, such as the name of the person who selects the health care plan, the ASLP health needs of the entity, and sources of ASLP health care the organization is currently using. With this information, a more effective presentation of the ASLP program's services can be made.

Each sales staff member is as valuable in maintaining relationships and providing information as in the selling of services. This is particularly true for ASLP programs within hospitals, which are dependent on referrals from physicians and other individuals. The role of the salesperson is to ensure that the program and its staff are meeting the referral sources' needs. If problems or areas of dissatisfaction are discovered, they should be brought to the attention of the program administrator, to be resolved immediately. And once resolved, it is very important to let consumers know of the improvement.

Another means of personal selling is to promote positive top-of-mind awareness among the physicians from whom you hope to receive referrals. By achieving name recognition and top-of-mind awareness, physician referrals will be made to your organization. The provider can solidify the relationship with referral sources in many ways. By thinking of the referring physician as a customer, program staff can promote a secure bond. Involve the referral source in the treatment team. This approach keeps the referral source informed, positions the referral source nicely with the patient, and definitely helps to solidify the relationship between the referral source and the provider. Frequent and appropriate communication with your referral sources is critical to maintaining good relationships. Program administrators should evaluate the program's attractiveness, business strengths, growth potential, vulnerability to competition, profitability, competitive intensity, and value as these issues relate to the consumer. In this instance, the term "value" refers to such amenities as hours of service, location, credit policy, reputation, scheduling system, telephone call follow-up, and other factors that tend to differentiate one competitor from another. All of these factors should be evaluated and the most appropriate mix chosen based upon the market being targeted by the personal selling effort.

Large health care organizations usually have separate programs for advertising and public relations. Often, however, some of that program's roles and responsibilities may be delegated to other individuals within the organization. It is important to ensure that these individuals' objectives are consistent with the organization's overall promotional plan. If different, confusion may result among the organization's consumers. In the absence of public relations and advertising professionals within the organization, the ability to reach target markets will require release time from clinical duties in order for the staff to accomplish the marketing objectives. Individuals tapped for public relations efforts must have high morale, ability, excellent communication skills, and a professional appearance if the desired image is to be properly communicated to the target audience.

Consumer Satisfaction

The ultimate goal in determining the marketing mix is to ensure customer satisfaction. Thus, customer satisfaction is an integral component of the marketing program (Swan, Sawyer, Van Matre, & McGee, 1985). What this means is the value of the customer as perceived by someone. What is meant is the customer's perception of value is the result of a comparison between service quality, price, and the other costs of acquiring the service. If performance exceeds expectations, the customer is highly satisfied. If performance meets expectations, the customer is usually satisfied. But if performance falls short of expectations, the customer will be dissatisfied.

Value, service quality, and costs are driven by employee retention and satisfaction. When employees are satisfied, customers generally report a higher level of satisfaction and remain customers. Profits are the outcome of employee and customer satisfaction and retention. Your customers can identify satisfying and dissatisfying employee behaviors, and their opinions should be taken seriously. The major challenge to an organization is not winning new customers, but retaining existing ones. Statistics show that customers who experience bad service complain to, on average, ten to twelve people, while those who experience good service tell only four or five people. Research (Hillestad & Berkowitz, 1991) has also shown that it is five times more expensive to attract a new customer than it is to retain an existing customer. Thus, the importance of customer satisfaction.

The ASLP programs can promote customer satisfaction in many ways. First of all, be straightforward about procedures and fees. Second, make sure the customer is aware of various treatment options, but state your treatment recommendations with conviction. Third, thoroughly train your office staff in the needs of the communicatively impaired. Fourth, follow up immediately with customers and referral sources after a visit to your organization. Fifth, send timely written reports to referral sources following diagnostic visits. Finally, ensure that services are offered at times and places convenient to the customers you wish to serve.

Customer satisfaction may be enhanced through attention to the extra touches that can help to distinguish a facility: clean reception areas, responsive call-backs, respect for the time constraints of others, assistance with filling out insurance forms, staff who call back after a day to make sure everything is all right, a birthday card, a quarterly newsletter

---

PATIENT SURVEY

We want to give you the best possible ASLP care during your visit. To do that we need your feedback. Your answers will be used to help us serve you better. This survey is completely voluntary, anonymous, and confidential. You do not need to sign the questionnaire. Please use this opportunity to respond. Thank you in advance.

ANSWER ALL QUESTIONS THAT APPLY TO YOU. CIRCLE ONE NUMBER FOR EACH QUESTION.

CLINIC RATING	VERY POOR	POOR	FAIR	GOOD	VERY GOOD
1. EASE OF GETTING AN APPOINTMENT	1	2	3	4	5
2. EASE OF GETTING TO THE CLINIC	1	2	3	4	5
3. COMFORT OF THE RECEPTION AREA	1	2	3	4	5
4. CLEANLINESS OF THE RECEPTION AREA	1	2	3	4	5
5. PROMPTNESS IN BEING SEEN	1	2	3	4	5
6. TELEPHONE COURTESY BY OUR STAFF	1	2	3	4	5
7. STAFF CONCERN FOR YOUR PRIVACY	1	2	3	4	5

CLINICAL CARE	VERY POOR	POOR	FAIR	GOOD	VERY GOOD
1. RECEIVED ADEQUATE ANSWERS TO YOUR HEARING/SPEECH QUESTIONS	1	2	3	4	5
2. SATISFACTION WITH THE QUALITY OF THE EVALUATION	1	2	3	4	5
3. CONFIDENCE AND TRUST IN YOUR CLINICIAN	1	2	3	4	5
4. ASLP's CARE FOR YOU	1	2	3	4	5
5. OVERALL RATING OF THE CLINIC	1	2	3	4	5

6. ARE YOU SCHEDULED TO COME BACK?   YES   NO

---

7. COMMENTS: _____

_____

_____

Figure 9–3. Sample patient survey.

about current topics, or a free bus ride for patients who are going to a downtown program. All these activities define the product or service offering and help determine how competitive it will be. Written patient surveys are probably the most popular method for obtaining feedback from patients. They may be given to patients at the time of their office visit, to be completed then or be returned in the mail. Sending the surveys by mail retains patient anonymity but is more expensive, especially if they are not returned. A sample of a customer survey is given in Figure 9–3. Patient surveys should be conducted continuously so that emerging trends may be identified as early as possible.

STEP 5: MARKETING ACTION PLAN

Once the marketing goals and objectives have been established and the marketing strategy developed, it is necessary to establish and implement specific actions intended to ensure achievement of the objectives. It is at this phase that marketing must act as a catalyst to help integrate the marketing plan into the overall business plan. The marketing action plan lists steps to be taken, in chronological order, along with starting date, target completion date, person responsible for the action, and estimated costs. A sample marketing plan (see Appendix 9A) describes the marketing tasks developed and implemented in order to accomplish the marketing objectives.

STEP 6: MARKETING BUDGET

The organization's convictions about the marketing effort will be tested by the dollars allocated to the effort. There are several means of allocating dollars to marketing. The most common way in which professional organizations determine their advertising budget is by calculating what they think they can afford (i.e., the affordable method). During the budgeting process, dollars are allocated to personnel, operations, capital improvements, new equipment purchases, and so forth. After the critical categories receive their allocated dollars, any "extra" monies are allocated to advertising. Programs that spend only "leftover" dollars on advertising tend to do so only because they think they should, not because of a conviction that it is money well spent. These organizations tend not to create specific objectives to direct the campaign. Nevertheless, the program administrator needs a starting point for the budget and this is not the most effective approach. Other approaches result in the more effective use of marketing dollars.

One of the most effective budgeting methods is the objective-based budget. It is based on the following steps: (1) define marketing objectives as specifically as possible; (2) determine the marketing tasks necessary to achieve each objective; and (3) estimate the cost of performing each marketing task. The sum of these costs determines the marketing budget. The advantage of having an objective-driven budget for marketing is that it allows for additional investment over time, should the need arise. Once the budgeting method to be used is decided, the marketing budget section of the marketing plan then summarizes anticipated costs associated with achieving the objectives.

STEP 7: INTEGRATION OF THE MARKETING PLAN

The marketing plan does not exist in isolation. Instead, it must be integrated with the functions of finance, personnel, and administrative operations within the health care organization (Clarke & Shyavitz, 1987; George & Compton, 1985; Miaoulis, Anderson, LaPlaca, Geduldig, Giesler, & West, 1985). Output from each of these functions provides input for the marketing plan and budget. The marketing data obtained in the foregoing steps serves as input into the plan and budget. When this process is carried out by each specialty within a program, it is likely that an imbalance in the budget will develop, with the result that the budget for each specialty (and thus, the marketing plan) within the program's total budget must be revised until a balance is reached. This process will ensure that competition within the program is minimized, resources are maximized, and the program is efficiently managed.

The process of integration is a dynamic one, based on personalities, politics, available resources, and the value system of the health care organization. Difficulty with the integration step can create the need for a revised marketing strategy, which may be different from the original strategy. Integration of the budgets is largely a mechanical task. It is done to determine if the necessary revenue and expense equalities exist. If they do, the marketing plan can be completed. If, however, an imbalance exists, then additional management judgment is needed.

STEP 8: MONITORING THE MARKETING PLAN

Monitoring the marketing plan is begun after its implementation to ensure that the desired results are achieved. Most monitoring actions have a short time span, and are designed to evaluate and modify marketing plans, if indicated. Regular monitoring of various practice parameters, such as sales, helps to determine what strategy should be used in future marketing plans. The monthly revenue and expense statement can be used to monitor sales by a specific specialty area. Table 9–1 shows total clinical procedures volume for the month, net income by ASLP evaluation, and the percentage return of profit for each dollar of services. This information shows those areas which generate strong profits for each dollar of services and those which are having difficulty. For example, ASLP procedure 4 demonstrates

Table 9–1. ASLP clinical procedures assessment.

PROCEDURE	TOTAL SERVICES $$	NET INCOME $$	PERCENTAGE RETURN ON SERVICES*
ASLP 1	3,000	2,000	67
ASLP 2	2,500	1,700	68
ASLP 3	2,000	1,300	65
ASLP 4	4,000	1,000	−25
*Return on services = $\frac{\text{Net income}}{\text{Services}}$			

Source: Adapted from *Health care marketing plans: From strategy to action* (2nd ed., p. 217) by S. G. Hillestad & E. N. Berkowitz, (1991), Gatlinburg, MD: Aspen Publisher, Inc.

increased services, but has a negative income. This type of information can be helpful in adjusting prices, eliminating services, or modifying the marketing plan to promote services in more promising areas.

Monitoring must be performed at regular intervals throughout the period of the marketing plan in order to check progress of key indicators against the marketing plan objectives. Any deviation from the expected, either better or worse than expected results, must be analyzed for the cause, and the marketing plan modified, if necessary.

PLANNING FOR THE FUTURE

Forecasting demand for each of the organization's respective service areas will be based on the current year's marketing and business plans. All projections are derived from current estimates of population growth for the service area by age, race, sex, income, and so forth, as previously discussed. These values, multiplied by clinician scheduling rates, will equal the total number of program visits to meet the service area demand by specialty. This type of information will help the organization refine its business direction and marketing strategies for future years.

CONCLUSION

The intent of this chapter has been to orient the ASLP administrator to the marketing environment and to build a foundation for examining these individual topics. The reader should have an improved understanding of the tools and techniques that can be of value in designing, implementing, and monitoring an effective marketing plan. The critical concept in this chapter is the active nature of marketing. Successful administrators are active in directing the public's awareness of their programs. These administrators continually evaluate the program's marketing performance and position themselves with an eye to enhancing strengths and correcting deficiencies.

REFERENCES

Aaker, D. A., & Shansby, J. C. (1982). Positioning your product. *Business Horizons, 25,* 56–62.

Abell, D. F., & Hammond, J. S. (1979). *Strategic market planning: Problems and analytical approaches.* Englewood Cliffs, NJ: Prentice-Hall.

Clarke, R. N., & Shyavitz, L. (1987). Health care marketing: Lots of talks, any action? *Health Care Management Review, 12,* 31–36.

George, W. R., & Compton, F. (1985). How to initiate a marketing perspective in a health care organization. *Journal of Health Care Marketing, 5,* 29–37.

Hillestad, S. G., & Berkowitz, E. N. (1991). *Health care marketing plans: From strategy to action* (2nd ed.). Gaithersburg, MD: Aspen.

Hunter, S. S. (1987). Marketing and strategic management: Integrating skills of a better hospital. *Hospital and Health Services Administration, 32,* 205–216.

Jensen, J. (1986). Health care alternatives. *American Demographics, 8,* 36–38.

Kotler, P. (1980). *Marketing management: Analysis, planning, and control.* Englewood Cliffs, NJ: Prentice-Hall.

MacStravic, R. S. (1988). Evaluating health care marketing. *Health Care Management Review, 13,* 45–57.

McDevitt, P. (1987). Learning by doing: Strategic marketing management in hospitals. *Health Care Management Review, 12,* 23–30.

Miaoulis, G., Anderson, D. C., LaPlaca, P. J., Geduldig, J. P., Giesler, R. H., & West, S. (1985). A model for hospital marketing decision processes and relationships. *Journal of Health Care Marketing, 5,* 37–45.

Nichols, P. (1986). Market oriented strategic planning, revisited. *Health Management Forum, 7,* 47–55.

Swan, J. E., Sawyer, J. C., Van Matre, J. C., & McGee, G. W. (1985). Deepening the understanding of hospital patient satisfaction: Fulfillment and equity effects. *Journal of Health Care Marketing, 5,* 7–18.

Weiss, R. (1990). Hitting the target. *Health Progress, 71,* 18–20.

Recommended Readings

Andreasen, A. R. (1982). Nonprofits: Check your attention to customers. *Harvard Business Review, 60,* 105–110.

Autrey, P., & Thomas, D. (1986). Competitive strategy in the hospital industry. *Health Care Management Review, 2,* 49–56.

Bloom, P. N. (1984). Effective marketing for professional services. *Harvard Business Review, 5,* 102–110.

Coile, R. C. (1989). Strategic marketing: 10 approaches that will work in the 1990s. *Hospital Strategy Report, 1,* 1–4.

Ferrell, O. C., Madden, C. S., & Legg, D. (1986). Strategic planning for nonprofit health care organization. *Journal of Health Care Marketing, 6,* 13–21.

Louden, T. L. (1989). Successful marketing plans for new products more important than ever. *Modern Health Care, 17,* 68.

APPENDIX 9A

Marketing Plan—Sample

Overview

The preparation of a marketing plan is a major duty of the program administrator. The following is a sample marketing plan for an ASLP program in Anywhere, USA. The purpose of this marketing plan is to assist the ASLP program to maintain quality of care, meet community needs, and ensure economic growth. This example is intended for use by the inexperienced program administrator in order to facilitate the preparation of a marketing plan. The steps of the marketing plan focus on the basic concepts disseminated in the marketing chapter.

In this scenario, the ASLP program did not meet its first year expectations due to inconvenient hours of operation and lack of community awareness. The program is planning to modify its operations to attract market segments that want convenience. It will also develop and implement a promotional program, and develop and implement new programs to encourage consumer trial use. If this strategy is effective, other specialties within the program will adopt similar strategies in order to boost recognition of the entire program. We describe the environment in terms of strengths and weaknesses of the program, the nature of the program's role within the community, the nature of the population being served, and the program's approach to marketing.

STEP 1: THE MARKETING MISSION

The mission of the ASLP program is to provide quality communication health care to a suburban community. Its goals are (1) to be a self-supporting group of clinicians, (2) to become the most sought after ASLP program in the surrounding community, (3) to provide a broad range of diagnostic and rehabilitative services, and (4) to generate a 10% return on investment.

STEP 2: ENVIRONMENTAL ASSESSMENT

Market Segmentation

Current patients include all age groups, with a heavy emphasis on the elderly and the very young. Men and women utilize the services of the program in equal numbers and most are in the middle to upper-middle income range. Few have third-party coverage. Furthermore, most patients come from within a 10-mile radius of the office.

Competition

There is one nonprofit clinic in the community that serves 15% of the available market through the efforts of one audiologist and three speech-language pathologists. The major advantages of the nonprofit clinic are its reasonably priced services, top-of-mind awareness in the community, and downtown location. Major disadvantages perceived by the market are high turnover of staff and difficulty in obtaining a timely appointment. Further competition comes from a two-person hearing aid practice that has been in the community for 30 years.

Internal Environment Assessment

This licensed and accredited ASLP program is one year old. The program is fully equipped to perform routine and specialized examinations. There are presently no maintenance costs; however, they can be expected to increase over the next 5 years. The program is presently utilized to 75% capacity and can accommodate additional markets.

The professional staff consists of 8 audiologists and 12 speech-language pathologists. A full range of inpatient and outpatient services is provided. The facility has been designated by the community as the primary provider of services for individuals with communication disorders. Operating agreements with local nursing facilities, home health care programs, and private corporations are in place. The community's lack of comprehensive communication health care resources indicates the potential for increased referrals of both pediatric and adult patients to this program. The program staff is well trained and sensitive to the needs of the organization, the community, patients, and referral sources. However, the staff is not satisfied with the current level of utilization of the service, or with the program's financial condition, due to less than anticipated first-year use. The program's geographic location affords high visibility as a result of the local traffic patterns. Competitors' locations are less than ideal in comparison.

External Environment Assessment

The population of this community is currently 100,000 persons; 20% of the population is enrolled in an HMO and obtains service in the metropolitan area. The population has remained relatively stable in size. The available pool of potential patients also appears satisfactory. However, the population has declined marginally in economic status while polarizing into two demographic groups; one aging and the other young, both of which are relatively unskilled. The number of referring physicians is currently 27.

The downturn in the economy has resulted in the elimination of many jobs locally and the scaling back of health care benefits. As a result, only 15% of all program visits are reimbursed by third-party payers. Forty percent of households are people living alone (single, separated, widowed, or divorced); 40% of all households have a husband and wife working; 65% of the local population is less than 55 years of age.

STEP 3: MARKETING GOALS AND OBJECTIVES

The primary strategy for the ASLP program is to continue to grow and to differentiate its services relative to those of the competition. The program has decided to enhance its reputation in the community by providing some new products and services. They will be made available to all community members regardless of economic status. It is hoped that the resulting increase in visibility and demonstration of concern for the community will increase the program's market share.

The marketing plan will attempt to achieve the following objectives: (1) increase patient visits from 7,500 this year to 9,000 by the end of the next fiscal year; (2) attempt to attract market segments seeking convenience, especially households where all adults are working, by offering evening and Saturday hours beginning April 1; (3) increase level of community awareness of the program from 60% to 75% of each of the target market segments by the end of the second quarter of the next fiscal year; (4) reach the break-even point by the end of the third quarter of the next fiscal year; and, (5) begin measuring customer satisfaction with regular use of customer satisfaction surveys.

STEP 4: MARKETING STRATEGY AND MARKETING ACTION PLAN

Product/Service Decisions

- Potential new products/services will be investigated as to the feasibility of their being offered. If feasible, they will be implemented.

Price Decisions

- Credit cards will be accepted in order to promote convenience and to enhance control of accounts receivable.
- Contracts with managed care plans will be explored as a means of increasing patient visits.
- Current customers will be offered a 10% discount each time they are named as a referral source by a new patient.
- Customers paying at the time of service will be given a 10% discount.

The program administrator is responsible for developing pricing strategies. The exact costs are to be determined. The expected outcome of the new pricing strategy is new patient volume, decreased accounts receivable, and increased income. Steps 1, 3, and 4 are to be completed in the 1st quarter; step 2 is to be completed in the 3rd quarter.

Place (Distribution) Decisions

The main strategy here is to establish new hours of operation in order to attract larger market segments. If this approach generates additional patient visits, the major growth element of this plan will be achieved.

- Program hours will be expanded from 9 a.m. to 9:30 p.m., Monday through Friday, and from 9 a.m. to 1 p.m. on Saturday, to attract and accommodate the working market.

Promotion Decisions

- Promotional materials will be developed which clearly explain the new program hours and scheduling procedures. Existing brochures will be distributed to the industrial organizations, senior citizen groups, and schools targeted for audiometric testing. This step will not result in additional cost to the service as this item is currently in the budget.

∎ A quarterly direct mail newsletter will be mailed to targeted households featuring short topics on communication disorders and the availability of services.

∎ A monthly statement stuffer will be sent to each patient with an outstanding balance, and will contain information about the program staff and its services.

∎ A computerized call-back system will be developed to remind patients of the need for reevaluations.

∎ Program visibility will be enhanced through monthly educational seminars to community organizations or public service groups. Staff members will be reimbursed their hourly wage for time spent at speaking engagements outside normal work hours, in addition to travel expenses. The cost of this step will not exceed $100 per month. Promotion will also include open houses and networking with other professionals who have contacts with the target market. The program administrator will assign promotional opportunities to appropriate staff members.

∎ Yellow Pages advertising will be evaluated by June 1, 1993, two months prior to the deadline for submitting ads. Current ads will be maintained or expanded, depending upon need. The program administrator will work closely with an outside advertising agency to evaluate the need for additional Yellow Pages advertising.

Step 1 will be completed in January; steps 2, 3, 4, and 5 are ongoing. An advertising agency and the program administrator will be responsible for developing printed promotional materials.

STEP 6: MARKETING BUDGET

The following marketing budget represents the program administrator's best estimate of the cost of initiating the ASLP marketing plan.
Marketing Budget for FY 1993–94:

1. Printed materials $8,000
2. Yellow Pages...1,500
3. Personal selling...2,700
4. Postage...550
5. Miscellaneous expenses 550

Total $13,300

Marketing expenses will not be increased by more than 2% during the next fiscal year. Each line item in the budget will be validated and expenses will be cut, when possible, in some areas. Line items which show greater than a 2% increase must be justified by a positive return on investment. The budget will be reviewed with the staff to evaluate alternatives to current expenditures. The program administrator will assume this responsibility and will meet regularly with the staff to discuss the marketing budget.

STEP 7: INTEGRATION OF THE MARKETING PLAN

Several members of the program staff will participate in implementation of the plan. The program administrator will be responsible for the overall plan. Each unit will be allocated marketing funds based on its goals and objectives.

STEP 8: MONITORING THE MARKETING PLAN

Once the marketing budget has been approved and implementation of the plan has begun, revenue and expense reports will be examined monthly. Should revenues fall short of the anticipated amount or should unexpected expenses arise, a marketing budget freeze may occur, or advertising expenditures may be cut. If the program fails to show substantial growth by the 3rd quarter, several options will be explored, including: (1) elimination of an ASLP specialty function within the program; (2) sale of the ASLP program to another group; or, (3) closure of the practice and sale of the facility.

10

CLOSING REMARKS

Stephen R. Rizzo, Jr., PhD and
Michael D. Trudeau, PhD

"*O*ne *of life's most painful moments comes when we must admit that we did not do our homework, that we are not prepared.*" (Merlin Olsen, NFL Commentator)

This is the second opportunity we as editors have to address you. In this book on clinical administration in ASLP, the contributors have shared with you their thoughts on some of the issues confronting us health care professionals.

Traditional education programs in ASLP and in health care administration are separated by barriers established over time. The educational spheres of each have become increasingly institutionalized, leading to a growing gap between the two when increasing overlap is needed. You, our readers, have taken your own personal steps in creating a bond between education and practice. We, as both clinicians and administrators, must lead the "ASLP evolution" toward formal educational patterns in administration. The question that must be addressed is, "How does one evolve to become an ASLP administrator?" The task is not a simple one, for ASLP administration is not a curriculum in itself. It is a multidisciplinary field including medicine, education, behavioral sciences, economics, and management. Hence, our organizational structure, cultural and ethnic diversity, academic objectives, and teaching methods are pertinent factors to analyze and modify if our academic programs are to educate the ASLP administrators of the future.

The administrative evolution among all ASLP participants (i.e, students, clinicians, teachers, and researchers) should be kept alive as a deep commitment in their professional lives. The ultimate goal is not to impart or teach content areas of administration, but rather to expose and stimulate clinicians, teachers, and researchers to be knowledgeable of the management of clinical, scientific, or public career opportunities they may wish to pursue.

The evolution from clinician to ASLP administrator is particularly important because of the current health care environment and the fact that the delivery of clinical services is being increasingly influenced by government regulations concerning cost, quality, and quantity of patient care. ASLP administrators must be good managers who utilize business-oriented methods and organizational goals to control the use of resources.

The absence of trained program administrators, and the growing leadership emphasis displayed by other professionals in allied health care organizations will influence ASLP policies and affect the way communication health care is organized and delivered. There is evidence that ASLPs are not receiving formal training in administration. A recent survey on ASLP administration (Rizzo, Gutnick, & Stein, 1992) revealed that in 125 university training programs surveyed, very few offered formal curriculum opportunities in administration. By better understanding the factors that influence ASLPs to become administrators, training programs may restructure their curricula to be of maximum vocational benefit to potential managers without compromising current quality of clinical education. This understanding could enhance ASLP organizations to improve the recruitment and retention of competent program administrators.

The influence of role models, preceptors, and teachers on the evolution to ASLP administrator has received little attention. Mentorship has been recognized as an important developmental tool for success (Abrams, 1991; Collins & Scott, 1978; Gibbons, 1992; Hunt & Michael, 1983; Kovach & Moore, 1992; Peters & Austin, 1985; Seymour, Stewart, & Tibbits, 1992; Shapiro, Haseltine, & Rowe, 1978; Zey, 1984). Mentors influence the psychosocial development of managers, promotion decisions, and the support and counsel of protégés who are "on the know and on the grow."

The importance of on-the-job experience in the growth and development of the program administrator has not appeared in the literature. Most ASLPs move into administrative positions without special training and learn administrative skills almost exclusively through experience. These individuals receive initial exposure to administration by observing their clinical supervisors in the management of an Audiology or Speech-Language Pathology section. This encounter may be the only opportunity to inspect administrative assignments prior to making a significant career decision. The first administrative assignment in the career of the ASLP is usually that of unit supervisor or section chief in either a hospital or outpatient setting. The administrative skills for these positions are generally acquired through supervised trial and error. Administrative experience obtained through on-the-job training, although influential, requires further scrutiny because it represents only one aspect of a multifaceted process.

A growing concern of some educators (Cunningham, Lingwall, Steckol, Baker, & Gore, 1981; Cunningham, 1992) is the need for teaching administration to ASLPs at the graduate training level. This training is a prerequisite for adapting to the increasing administrative demands of management in a complex health care environment. While knowledge of these issues is included in formal administration and leadership training workshops, it would be beneficial to identify those aspects of training which are associated with positive outcomes versus those aspects associated with less effective administrative outcomes. The impetus for the professional doctorate degree will place more emphasis on program performance and results. To achieve this, university programs need to integrate administrative theory into the ASLP training program. In addition, consideration should be given to incorporating an administrative component into the practicum and the clinical fellowship year (CFY) experience (focusing on management theory, business methods, and supervised administrative experiences).

In closing, this book has focused on the role of an administrator at the director or manager level. We hope that we have raised more questions than answers. This is obviously a process in which one plants the seeds, cultivates the land, and hopes for a good crop. As General George S. Patton once said, "Accept the challenges so that you may feel the exhilaration of victory."

REFERENCES

Abrams, H. B. (1991, September). Framework for management development. Paper presented at the Task Force Planning Meeting on Problem-Based Treatment Outcome Measurement. Department of Veterans Affairs, Alexandria, VA.

Collins, E., & Scott, P. (1978). Everyone who makes it has a mentor. *Harvard Business Review, 56,* 89–101.

Cunningham, D. R., Lingwall, J. B., Steckol, K. F., Baker B. M., & Gore, L. B. (1981). Professional issues curriculum for audiology and speech-language pathology. *Asha, 23,* 885–897.

Cunningham, D. R. (1992). Personal communication.

Gibbons, A. (1992). Key issue: Mentoring. *Science, 255,* 1368.

Hunt, D. M., & Michael, C. (1983). Mentorship: A career training and developmental tool. *Academy of Management Review, 8,* 475–485.

Kovach, T. M., Moore, S. M. (1992). Leaders are born through the mentoring process. *Asha, 34,* 33–35.

Peters, T., & Austin, N. (1985). *A passion for excellence: The leadership difference.* New York: Random House.

Rizzo, S. R., Gutnick, H. N., & Stein, D. W. (1992). Survey of audiology and speech-language pathology university training programs: Preparation in administration. Unpublished manuscript.

Seymour, C. M., Stewart, B. A., & Tibbits, D. F. (1992). Mentoring fosters leadership. *Asha, 34*, 45–47.

Shapiro, E. C., Haseltine, F. P., & Rowe, M. P. (1978). Moving up: Role models, mentors and the patron system. *Sloan Management Review, 19*, 51–58.

Zey, M. (1984). *The mentor connection.* Homewood, IL: Irwin.

INDEX